HOW TO BEAT CHRONIC LYME

THROUGH PHYSICAL, EMOTIONAL & SPIRITUAL HEALING

ROBERT GROLEAU

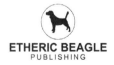

ETHERIC BEAGLE
PUBLISHING

How To Beat Chronic Lyme Through Physical, Emotional &
Spiritual Healing
Copyright © 2015 by Robert Groleau.

Robert Groleau/Etheric Beagle Publishing
2918 Ranch Rd 620 N, #240
Austin, Texas 78734
www.robertgroleau.com
E-mail: robert@robertgroleau.com

Cover Design by Robert Groleau
Book Layout ©2013 BookDesignTemplates.com
Editing by Sally Hanan, www.inksnatcher.com

Publisher's Cataloging-in-Publication data

Names: Groleau, Robert.
Title: How to beat chronic Lyme through physical , emotional & spiritual
healing / Robert Groleau.
Identifiers: ISBN 978-0-9971458-0-9 | LCCN 2015921083.
Description: Austin [Texas] : Etheric Beagle Publishing, 2016 | Includes
bibliographical references.
Subjects: LCSH Lyme Disease--Treatment. | Lyme disease--Alternative
treatment--United States. | Holistic medicine. | Spiritual healing. | Mind
and body. | BISAC HEALTH & FITNESS / Diseases / General.
Classification: LCC RC155.5 .G76 2016 | DCC 616.9/2—dc23

Disclaimer: This publication is sold with the understanding that the author is not engaged in rendering medical or psychological services. This
book is not intended as a substitute for the medical advice of physicians,
or the counseling of therapists. If expert assistance is needed, the services of a competent physician or therapist should be sought.

To my parents, who set the stage for the healing journey of a lifetime, which is exactly what I needed.

Contents

Preface

I had Lyme disease for twenty-five years without knowing it. In 2001 I got bitten by a tick, which caused another Lyme infection. This began my long healing journey. This book is a description of the fourteen-year journey I took to overcome chronic Lyme disease, starting in 2001. I spent the first ten years receiving physical healing (the first two-and-a-half years in conventional medicine, then switching to alternative medicine after that). Then I spent three years receiving emotional healing, and I spent the most recent year, 2015, learning the spiritual concept of nonresistance, which is essential to the healing process. Of course, the physical healing work has continued all through each phase.

I discovered, after ten years, that when my physical healing reached an impasse, it was necessary to move into emotional healing to work on the underlying causes of the illness in order to get my physical healing back on track. What I discovered on this journey has been put into this book for the purpose of helping others to recover from this illness. Emotional healing is a big area to get into, and navigate. Most people don't know much about it, and don't think they need to know. The only option of treatment that most are aware of is costly long-term therapy, so I have provided an overview of the whole process, what I learned in it, and how to go about it. I have pulled together the best resources that helped me and presented them here.

While I have provided a lot of information in "Part I - Physical Healing," I believe the biggest acceleration you will find on your healing path will come from "Part II - Emotional Healing" and "Part III - Spiritual Healing."

— Robert Groleau

Introduction

This book is broken down into three parts representing the three phases of healing I went through, plus a conclusion. At the beginning of each part, I describe my personal story and then go on to a discussion of issues. I have included a list of helpful resources at the end of each part.

Part I - Physical Healing describes my journey using conventional and alternative medicine modalities in the treatment of chronic Lyme disease. You can save yourself a great deal of trouble by avoiding treating Lyme disease with medications that harm the gut flora—the beneficial bacteria in the intestines. If you cannot avoid this and have harmed your gut flora, as I did, then this book will help describe how to work your way through chronic illness.

Part II - Emotional Healing explains how you form emotional issues, how they affect your health, how to spot them, and how to work on healing them. It explains why Lyme disease patients share similar emotional issues. If emotional issues are the root cause of illness, then emotional healing may be the best thing you can do to move your physical healing forward.

Part III - Spiritual Healing discusses the concept of non-resistance. Suffering on a daily basis due to severe illness causes huge emotional resistance. This resistance creates more emotional issues which block your body's ability to heal itself. You are not aware you are doing this or of the effects it causes. Even if you were, how do you stop suffering from illness? Effective tools are provided to clear these blocks, which will facilitate healing.

Conclusion sums up the book.

This book is not a scientific treatise on all the technical aspects of this illness. I am describing my experiences with this illness and what I learned from my perspective. There are suggestions on how to cope with this illness, and how to maintain your physical and emotional health based on what I have learned from alternative health sources. I am not a doctor, nor a psychotherapist. I am not giving medical advice or counseling. None of this discussion should take the place of proper medical care by a physician. This book is my practical description of issues and treatments that helped me recover my health, written in layman's terms.

PART I

PHYSICAL HEALING

[1]

What Is Chronic Lyme Disease?

LYME DISEASE

Lyme disease is an illness caused by the bacteria Borrelia burgdorferi, which is typically transmitted by the bite of infected ticks. This infection often comes with bacteria that cause coinfections such as Ehrlichia, Babesia and Bartonella. These are the known coinfections.

CHRONIC ILLNESS

A chronic illness is a condition that lasts for a very long time, and it usually cannot be cured completely. In some cases it can be controlled.

CHRONIC VERSUS ACUTE LYME DISEASE

Lyme disease is considered acute or chronic depending on the amount of time that has passed since the initial infection, typically, but not always, from a tick bite. If it is a recent infection, it is considered acute. If it is a long-term infection, it is considered chronic.

If you get a new Lyme infection and treat it within about ten days with a short course of antibiotics, you can eradicate it completely. A longer term chronic infection is different. The Lyme bacteria have learned how to survive in your body over time. As you acquire other health issues, these issues can help to shield Lyme bacteria from treatment, so a longer course of treatment may be required.

The Lyme bacteria themselves create biofilms which protect them from treatment. Mercury in the body can also help shield bacteria from treatment. So chronic illness not only adds additional health issues to deal with, but the additional issues make the Lyme disease more resistant to treatment, and long-term treatment can weaken the immune system.

THE DOWNWARD SPIRAL OF LYME DISEASE INTO CHRONIC ILLNESS

- The Lyme infection overwhelms the immune system.
- A compromised immune system can no longer manage many of the health issues in the body that have previously been held in check.

- Treating Lyme disease with medications that harm the gut flora further weakens the immune system.
- The destruction of gut flora and the weakening of the immune system facilitate the growth of Candida, a fungus that spreads all over the body.
- As the body weakens and the immune system is compromised, pathogens multiply. The body becomes more toxic, which overloads the lymphatic system and elimination channels.
- The digestive system develops dysfunction. Parasites thrive and chew holes through the intestines, causing leaky gut syndrome—where food particles go through holes in the intestines into the bloodstream. There, they cause allergic reactions and autoimmune responses—where the body starts attacking itself.
- With digestive dysfunction and damaged gut flora your body does not digest and assimilate food, vitamins and minerals well, making it difficult for the body to get proper nutrition.
- From here, it's a downward spiral of health into chronic illness even if you can eliminate the Lyme infection.

THE SITUATION WITH CHRONIC LYME

This book is not about acute Lyme. That case is straightforward, as mentioned above. This book is about having chronic Lyme—when many courses of antibiotics have not eliminated the illness, and there is no clear path forward. It is also about the chronic illness issues that develop during the course of treatment. In my case, I got over Lyme disease in 2005, but because I had done severe damage to my gut flora, which undermined my immune system, I then had a whole range of significant chronic health issues caused by that. It took me another ten years to resolve those issues after overcoming Lyme.

How Did We Get Chronic Lyme Disease?

Many people, including myself, got a Lyme infection without knowing it, and they suffered many symptoms they just lived with for many years because nobody could diagnose it. At some point a Lyme disease diagnosis is made by a doctor and then treatment begins. So where are you when treatment begins? Do you already have other health issues? Have you discovered the Lyme infection shortly after getting it or did it occur years ago? Every person has a different combination of circumstances, but as mentioned previously, Lyme disease and various health issues can combine to ruin your health. Typical conventional treatment involves antibiotics, which may be long term, depending on the doctor and the severity of the case.

What To Do When Treatment Fails?

It is after long-term antibiotic treatment, when the illness has not been eliminated, that many people find themselves, and they don't know what to do next. Many turn to alternative medicine. Whichever road you take, it is no easy path, as your gut flora has been damaged and your immune system compromised.

Having a chronic illness can mean you have dozens of different health issues in addition to the Lyme infection. Some are fungi, bacteria, viruses, toxins, parasites, leaky gut syndrome, a weak immune system, allergies, and nervous system issues. Even if you can eliminate the Lyme infection, you then have to resolve all these other issues to recover your health. Recovery not only means killing pathogens, it also means healing all of your body's systems and bringing them back into balance once the pathogens are gone. In many cases it took years to throw your body's systems out of balance. Getting them back in balance will take time as well.

This book is about the path I took through these issues to recover from chronic Lyme disease over a fourteen-year period after the Lyme disease diagnosis. Before that, I had Lyme disease for twenty-five years without knowing it.

[2]

My Story - 2001 to 2015

2001 - TICK BITE IN TEXAS

On May 24, 2001, I was inspecting an old truss bridge in Goldthwaite, Texas. I finished and realized I had to cross a wooden fence to get back to my truck. I could see the fence was weak. If I'd stepped on the crossbeam to climb over, it would have broken. The landowner was outside mowing his lawn and I didn't want to create an incident, so I decided to roll on the ground under the wooden crossbeam of the fence. When I got back to my truck, I could see that I had a few ticks on me. I pulled them off as best I could and finished the rest of my workday. When I got back to the hotel, I showered. Afterward, I did a further examination of my body and found two ticks around my navel. I got some tweezers and pulled them off, but I grabbed the ticks by the body. The squeezing force of the tweezers squirted all of the tick's body contents into me. I was concerned but hoped for the best. The next day I finished work on my job and drove home for Memorial Day weekend.

Lyme Symptoms

The following day, Saturday, I couldn't get off the couch all day due to fatigue. The same thing happened on Sunday, so that week I went to see my local doctor in Austin, Texas. He looked right at the Lyme rash near my navel and said, "I see the rash, but there is such a low incidence of Lyme disease in Texas that I don't think you have Lyme." Well, I did some research online and found that there was not a low incidence of Lyme disease in Texas. The official Lyme disease count was low, but that's because it was either misdiagnosed or not reported properly. I did find out that if you get a new Lyme infection and treat it within ten days of the tick bite with a course of antibiotics, you can wipe it out completely.

The Search for Quick Treatment

The clock was ticking now on my ten-day window, and I had already used up several days. I had seen a doctor and that hadn't helped at all, and he could offer no further help. Now I was on my own and stress was building. I read about doctors who specialize in Lyme disease, called Lyme-literate MDs (LLMDs), and I found one in Dallas. I drove to Dallas and quickly got antibiotics. The doctor put me on a thirty-day course of the antibiotic Doxycycline. Having begun a course of antibiotics within ten days, I was relieved that I had nipped Lyme disease in the bud. I had done a lot of research, there was a lot of stress given the time constraint, and I had to drive three hours to Dallas, but I got the job done. That was a relief, and I was glad I would not have to drive back to Dallas again just to see a doctor.

I did the thirty-day course of antibiotics. The day I stopped taking the antibiotics, I got a severe pain in the arch of my foot. I didn't think much of it, but I did remember having that same pain in my foot one other time in my life, back in 1975.

1975 - CONNECTICUT

I grew up in Hamden, Connecticut, which is about an hour west of Old Lyme, Connecticut, where Lyme disease started in 1975.

PLUM ISLAND

In the book *Lab 257*, by Michael Christopher Carroll, the origins of Lyme disease are discussed as coming from a germ warfare laboratory on Plum Island, which is an island in the Long Island Sound directly across from the town of Old Lyme. The lab was run by an ex-Nazi named Erich Traub, known for infected tick experiments on human populations. The author traced bird and insect migration routes from Long Island up through Old Lyme. It is suspected that infected livestock used in tick experiments were carelessly left outside, and birds and insects feeding off the livestock brought the tick infections up through Old Lyme in 1975, where it was contracted by humans.[1] It's interesting information, but knowing it does not help anyone get over the illness.

Strange Foot Pain in Summer of 1975

So in the summer of 1975, when I was fourteen years old and living in Connecticut, I developed a mysterious symptom. I would get a very severe, but intermittent, sharp pain on the bottom of my feet. I was athletic, so this was noticeable. I can remember having a conversation with my baseball coach one day while walking off the field after a game, when I was struck by a sudden severe pain in my foot and couldn't walk. I had to sit down and have someone look at it, but minutes later the pain was completely gone. I may have had other symptoms, but I don't remember. The foot pain would come and go all summer, and then it stopped completely. Lyme disease was in the news, but no doctors considered it yet. Nobody could diagnose my foot problem. My doctor told me the foot pain was probably just due to growing pains.

Mysterious Symptoms over the Years

Over the years I suffered from depression and mysterious health issues. The depression started around age fifteen and continued intermittently. I have always had digestive issues since then. In my thirties I would get bouts of severe nausea that would come one day every month. This would go on for several consecutive months before vanishing suddenly. My neck became very stiff and stayed that way. I would get bouts of severe fatigue at various times, but not that often. However, these seemingly unrelated symptoms were not enough for an illness diagnosis by doctors. After years of seeking medical help and having doctors thinking I was imagining all this, I just learned to live with these issues.

2001 - CONTINUATION OF TEXAS LYME EPISODE

CONTINUED SYMPTOMS

The symptoms continued after my first round of Doxycycline ended, so I had to keep taking antibiotics. And I had to start making monthly drives to the doctor in Dallas, but at least I was finally solving this problem. Lyme disease can be sexually transmitted, and I found out I had given my wife a case of Lyme disease as well, so she started treatment with me. As time went on, it became more and more evident that I had had Lyme disease for a long time, perhaps many years. Eventually we put all the pieces together and realized it had actually started in 1975. I had had Lyme disease for about twenty-five years without knowing it or treating it. I was now forty years old.

So the pieces of the puzzle were now coming together. The many mysterious health symptoms I had had for decades were now starting to make sense.

CONVENTIONAL LYME DISEASE TREATMENT

During the next two-and-a-half years, I did constant courses of some of the most powerful antibiotics available. I would drive to Dallas from my home in Austin once a month for doctors' visits, hoping that each visit would be the last. I did courses of Doxycycline, Amoxicillin, Biaxin, Zithromax, Levaquin, and others. I took an unusual prescription liquid drug for Babesia that cost $1,000 per month. The Babesia infection was probably worse than the Lyme. Every month I would get a bout of nausea so severe that I would sometimes pass out while sitting with my head in the toilet, and wake up some time later on my back on the bathroom floor. Still, I continued on with life as if all was progressing. We enjoyed traveling, so in September of 2001 my wife and I traveled to London and Paris. The illness was starting to affect the traveling, but I could still do it.

The treatment and doctors' appointments continued. By 2003, I was doing heavy doses of Biaxin, Zithromax, and Amoxicillin in combination. By this time it was apparent that I had chronic Lyme that was resistant to treatment. I was still trying to live a normal life, but it was starting to appear that things were not improving. We took a trip to Spain in September. I caught a bad cold on the trip which would not go away, and I had to see a doctor to get more antibiotics. There was a great deal of fatigue on that trip. The traveling wasn't fun anymore. It was coming to an end.

TRYING TO GET OFF ANTIBIOTICS

In the fall of 2003, my Lyme disease was under control, so I tried to go off antibiotics. When a Lyme blood test would say that the Lyme was gone, I stopped taking antibiotics; however, the Lyme disease would then quickly return. So I got back on antibiotics. My LLMD was working with an alternative medicine practitioner who was recommending supplements for immune support. I took a colostrum supplement and some other products for a while. After a month or two I tried to go off antibiotics again. But the Lyme returned quickly. I got back on antibiotics and then went through the same process of trying to get off them a few more times.

BAD NEWS

At the end of 2003, it was apparent that I was not able to get off antibiotics. I was taking heavy doses of multiple powerful antibiotics to try to knock the Lyme out, but it wasn't working. One day, my LLMD in Dallas told me that it was time to stop treatment and learn to just accept my illness. Medicine could do no more for me. I was devastated. I hadn't seen that coming.

NEW RESOLVE

I recall driving home from that appointment with no hope. I had always believed in modern medicine. *The US has the best health care system in the world. This was the best science could offer?*, I thought. I had put my faith in doctors my whole life, and it had always worked out well. Now, medicine had abandoned me. I got home and took a shower. I remember standing there in the running water, and it came to me:

If no doctor could solve my illness, then I'll solve it myself.

From that day onward I became a research machine. I was determined to solve this problem and recover my life. Even though I was in miserable health and was getting only a few hours of sleep per night, I was still able to do my job inspecting bridges. It made a good income, so I had the funds to do whatever research and treatment I wanted. My life became a research project. I could only see a doctor for about one hour per month, but I had to live with this illness 24/7, so I became my own top medical advisor and did my own research. From then on, while I listened to doctors and practitioners, I was making the final decisions on my health using the knowledge and wisdom I had acquired. My days of putting my health in the hands of others, and trusting them completely, were over. This is my body. I make the decisions for this body.

2004 - THE MOVE TO ALTERNATIVE MEDICINE

A practitioner I know informed me that he was working with an alternative medicine doctor named Yoshiaki Omura, MD from Japan. He had a method of testing that involved a laser, substance samples, and muscle testing. It was fascinating. He still prescribed pharmaceutical medicines, but he stimulated acupuncture meridians to increase the uptake of the drugs to specific places in the body where they were needed. That was my first foray into alternative medicine, about which I knew very little. It was interesting, but didn't help me all that much.

DR. COWDEN

In early 2004, I heard of Dr. Lee Cowden, MD, a leading specialist in alternative medicine. Dr. Cowden is a cardiologist who went into alternative medicine to work with chronic illnesses. He used kinesiology at the time, testing many substance samples for resonance with the body. He would test for many things: Lyme, other bacteria, viruses, toxins, parasites, allergies, the effect of EMFs (electromagnetic fields), and more. This was the first I knew of all these types of issues affecting health. Dr. Cowden would recommend supplements and other alternative treatments for these issues. His protocols were extensive in an attempt to address as many issues as possible. He also prescribed energetic treatments to detoxify the body of the toxins and chemicals which interfere with the immune system. As alternative medicine is not covered by insurance, the protocols were expensive. Lyme disease is not a poor person's illness. The cost of conventional medicine treatment for Lyme disease is very expensive, and alternative medicine is not much better. The reason many people stick with conventional medicine treatment is because it is covered by insurance.

HERBAL LYME TREATMENT

We discovered that the antibiotics had knocked out the second Lyme infection that I acquired in 2001, but that the original Lyme infection was still there after twenty-five years, despite the recent antibiotic treatment. Dr. Cowden recommended Samento, an antibacterial herb by

Nutramedix as the main treatment for Lyme. It worked quite well, and it does not harm gut flora. This herb was working as well as all the powerful antibiotics I had been taking earlier; however, whenever I would try to go off the Samento, the Lyme disease would come back. My immune system was not strong enough to take over after quitting the medicine. Still, there was no harm to the body in taking the Samento since it did not harm gut flora.

During this time we discovered that my wife had overcome her bout with Lyme, as she did not have the long-term case of it that I had.

LYME & BODY TEMPERATURE

Lyme bacteria require a cooler body temperature than normal to survive. The bacteria actually lower your body temperature to accommodate themselves. My body temperature was always around 96° F when I had Lyme, as opposed to the normal 98.6° F. I experimented with hot baths to kill the bacteria, but I could only stand baths up to 110° F, and it was just not hot enough to heat the interior of the body to a point where it would affect the Lyme bacteria.

PARASITES

Right from the beginning of my treatment with Dr. Cowden, it became apparent that parasites were as much of a problem as Lyme, and maybe even more so. Parasites in humans are either worms or protozoa. Worm types are either flatworms, flukes or roundworms. Protozoa are microscopic single-celled organisms. I had all of them, but the biggest problem was that I had a severe infestation of Ascaris Lumbricoides, which is a type of roundworm that can grow to be 14 inches in length. My case was so extensive that no treatment had any effect. I could feel the parasites painfully burrowing through my organs, and my mood was constantly irritable. I had not yet figured out that it was helpful to give up sugar, which is parasites' favorite food. I remember in early 2005 taking the drug Albendazole for the parasites, and its effect was miraculous. All the parasites instantly disappeared. My body was quiet and peaceful, and my attitude was happy. I was thrilled. However, two weeks later more parasite eggs had hatched, and it was no different than before. I took Albendazole again, only this time it was about half as effective as before. Parasites can mutate and learn how to develop resistance to treatments. The third time I used Albendazole, it had almost no effect. The miracle drug no longer worked, and my hope for eliminating parasites and feeling better was crushed. It was back to herbs, which were not having much effect. Dr. Cowden told me that I had probably the worst case of parasites he had seen.

RIFE MACHINE USE

I spent a great deal of time working with a Rife machine to kill parasites and fungus. A Rife machine delivers electromagnetic energy at specified frequencies. When you match the frequencies that the parasites operate at, resonance occurs and the parasites are killed. I did a great deal of research and experimentation with the Rife machine. I used expanding and contracting ranges of frequencies to help keep parasites from mutating away from the frequencies that would kill them. The Rife machine was quite effective at killing parasites, but it could not eliminate them. Nothing else was working either though.

DENTAL WORK

Dr. Cowden made it clear that mercury was a big issue with chronic Lyme disease. I found a good biological dentist and had all my fillings removed and replaced with nonmetallic materials that were tested to be more compatible with my body. I also read a book called *The Root Canal Cover Up* by George Meinig, in which he explained that root canals harbor toxins which continue to drip into your body every day for the rest of your life—another toxic load that your immune system needs to handle.[2] So I also had my root canals removed. All this work cost about $10,000.

DIET CHANGE

I switched to a full vegetarian diet sometime in 2004, and continued that for three years, after which I did it on and off for a few more years. It never helped with parasites. I have tried several diets for health. They all have some good points. None are perfect.

I began to eliminate sugar from my diet. It was difficult at first. I would stop for a while and then binge on a box of donuts, but the punishment was always severe. I would feel miserable after eating sugar due to the parasites and Candida. Over time the brief pleasure of eating sugar was outweighed by the misery of the hours of suffering that followed. It took a long time before that logic had sunk in enough for me to resist eating sweets altogether. Eventually, I was able to walk by the donut section in the grocery store and not be tempted, though during the holidays I still could not resist the plates of cookies sitting around everywhere. Eventually, I came to resist even that. It probably took about three years to completely overcome the urge to eat sugar.

MORGELLON'S SYMPTOMS

In 2005, I went through something similar to Morgellon's disease. I was finding a few thin white filaments coming out of my skin, though not many. I also had the feeling that insects were biting my legs when I was lying down, but there were no actual bugs. That went on for months. I still have no idea what it was. It may have been related to parasites. In any case, it went away after some time. My body was just a merry-go-round of new symptoms, one phase after another.

ENDLESS SEARCH FOR PRACTITIONERS

I have found that no one practitioner can handle the many issues of chronic illness. There are too many issues, too many testing methods, and too many treatments for any one person to be able to handle it all. Sometimes one practitioner can handle an issue really well for a while, but to finish it off, another practitioner is better suited. So I kept an open mind and was always on the lookout for the next practitioner who could help me. Dr Cowden's knowledge and skills covered a lot of ground, but I still worked with other practitioners if I thought it could benefit me.

TREATMENT FOR ASCARIS

As mentioned previously, I had a severe infestation of the parasite Ascaris lumbricoides. In late 2005, I did some research on Hulda Clark's work with parasites (see chapter 4 for details). She was a well-known naturopath. I found an interesting treatment for Ascaris lumbricoides using ozonated olive oil. Well, I tried it, and the effect was horrific but spectacular. The die-off felt like the sensation of pins and needles when your foot falls asleep—kind of unbearable, but it is only in your foot and it only lasts for twenty seconds. The die-off of the extensive roundworm infection I had was like pins and needles all over my body, only it lasted for about four hours. Standing, sitting, lying down, moving, being still, rolling on the floor . . . none of it helped. There was no way to ease the suffering for four hours, and at the time, I did not know when it would end. It just seemed like endless suffering. I felt good afterwards though. This was only the beginning of my journey with parasites, but until then nothing had been able to put a dent in the roundworm infestation that had riddled my body. Dr. Cowden was shocked the next time I saw him, as nothing had worked with the roundworm before.

Unfortunately I had many types of parasites, so this breakthrough was just the very beginning.

BATHTUB METAPHOR FOR CHRONIC ILLNESS

As for the entire process of healing the body from chronic illness, Dr. Cowden describes it using the metaphor of a bathtub full of dirty water which has several clogged drains, several faucets pumping in dirty water, and several closed clean water faucets. The trick is to open the clogged drains, which represent the elimination channels of the body: the lymphatic system, liver, kidneys, and bowels. Then the faucets pumping dirty water must be turned off. These represent processed foods, GMOs, pesticides, pathogens, toxins, EMFs, heavy metals, etc. Then the faucets pumping in clean water must be turned on. These represent clean water, healthy food, relaxation, exercise, etc. Once you begin to do all these things, you still have a bathtub filled with filthy water, but over time the water will become clearer and clearer, until one day it is all clear.

2006 - OVERCOMING THE LYME INFECTION

By the end of 2005, the Lyme infection was still there but under control. I had been taking the herb Samento for Lyme disease for two years. Samento is an antibacterial herb that does not harm gut flora. The use of antibiotics, and recently the herb Samento, had diminished the Lyme infection, but my immune system was too weak to control the Lyme disease on its own. I was not able to go off the Samento without Lyme disease returning. That was alright, as the Samento was not harming my gut flora, but I was not moving forward.

Laser Acupuncture Treatment

In mid-December 2005, I saw a new practitioner who had developed a treatment that was able to energetically program the body for the inverse energy of the Lyme bacteria using a laser infusion of the energy into the body through acupuncture points. Theoretically, the inverse energy of the bacteria would repel the energy of the actual bacteria, forcing the actual physical bacteria to leave the body. The treatment worked. I was able to stop taking the Samento without Lyme disease returning after that one treatment. (That practitioner has since retired, and he took that treatment method with him into retirement.)

Beyond Lyme

By early 2006, I no longer took any medication for Lyme disease; however, with chronic illness there were many health issues remaining. I stopped seeing Dr. Cowden in 2006 when he moved, and I just kept dealing with the issues that came up, finding new practitioners to handle them. I would stay with practitioners as long as their treatments were working for me. The biggest issue was the parasites, but there were many others. Many practitioners claimed their parasite treatments were the greatest ever and would definitely work for me. They were always wrong.

The practitioner with the energy treatment that helped me with Lyme had also treated me for parasites. His treatment did something that really helped. I was feeling better for a while. Having eliminated Lyme, and now really making progress on parasites, I thought I was getting close to the end of my illness. I felt there was finally a light at the end of the tunnel, and this long five-year illness nightmare was finally coming to an end. I wanted to travel again, and I scheduled a trip to Ecuador and Peru. My wife and I hadn't traveled in three years.

CHEMTRAILS

As it turned out, however, the parasites were only temporarily knocked back. They were not gone, and I discovered a new health issue—chemtrails. My practitioner told me about them and kept testing me for them. They can be determined easily with energy testing. You can test the person for them. You can test materials from outdoors. You can also test a photograph of the sky, as photographs capture energy. He could treat the chemtrails, but as soon as the skies were sprayed again I would feel bad. So just around the time I had overcome Lyme and was making progress on parasites, I found I had a new issue to overcome that was caused by people spraying chemicals in the sky. The day that I came to that realization, I was devastated; there was nothing I could do about it. It was back to feeling helpless again. The reason I was affected by chemtrails was because my immune system was weak. Over time, as my immune system strengthened, the chemtrails no longer affected me. In the meantime, I used homeopathics to detoxify them from my system.

Gallstones & Liver Flushes

We still traveled to Ecuador and Peru. I remember having some digestive issues while in Ecuador, so one day I went to a local health clinic on a street corner. They did a full range of parasite testing. The doctor also had a hunch and gave me an ultrasound test and found gallstones. Then he gave me an hour consultation on gallbladder surgery. The bill for all those services, after spending about four hours in his clinic, was $18.

When we returned from the trip, I saw my doctor (MD in Austin) about gallstones. He recommended I have my gallbladder surgically removed. I declined and began research on gallstones. The best option seemed to be liver flushes. I found a method I liked in a book called *The Amazing Liver and Gallbladder Flush*, by Andreas Moritz. I began the process in late 2006. As per the book, I thought a dozen flushes was the upper limit to clear stones out of the gallbladder. In a discussion with the author of the book, he informed me that people with certain emotional issues tend to constantly manufacture gallstones, and they get caught in the gallbladder. So even if you flush the stones out, you will just create more. I was one of those people. I wound up doing many more than a dozen flushes. As of 2015, I have done seventy-nine liver flushes. There was never any need to have my gallbladder removed. The flushes served as maintenance. I flushed some stones out of my gallbladder, but more were created and moved in there. I flushed out a lot of stones directly from my liver. I was later informed by a medical intuitive that as the liver is greatly affected by anger, a large amount of fatty material in the liver that holds anger issues is also flushed out during a liver flush. Liver flushes were one of the few treatments that directly led to my feeling better during my illness. The liver is aptly named—it makes you live. Keeping it clean is essential, especially in chronic illness when the body is dealing with such a heavy toxic load.

COLONICS & CLEANSING

Working on my diet because of gallstones, and dealing with the never-ending parasite issues took up most of my focus in 2007 and 2008. Around this time I became interested in colon hydrotherapy as a way to work on the digestive tract. If you have chronic illness, and especially if you have parasites, the colon can become a mess. Parasites back things up in the colon so that they can set up a comfortable refuge in there to lay eggs. Also, your body's other elimination channels may be backing up with toxins from chronic illness. It's important to keep the elimination channels moving at any time, but especially with chronic illness when they get overworked. I started doing colonics with a practitioner. I did a few weeklong fasting cleanses over time. Your body uses a lot of energy to digest food. If you stop eating, your body can rest and use the energy for elimination and detoxification during a fasting cleanse. On a supervised cleanse with a practitioner, you take supplements and drink fluids to maintain your health while fasting. Doing colonics every day during the cleanse helps elimination. After some time, I discovered home colonic kits online, and purchased one. I began to do colonics by myself at home. They are especially good with a liver flush, because you can clean out all the stones flushed from the liver. Otherwise, the stones can get hung up in the intestines and can cause discomfort.

2009 - Starting to Feel Better

My wife and I did not travel again after 2006. We divorced in 2008, and I started to feel better in 2009. Those two things are not unrelated. If you are in a relationship that is not working, it can harm your health. So after eight years of illness, I started feeling better and I went on my first trip in three years (in January of 2009) to visit the Mayan ruins in Mexico. I had stopped traveling due to the health issues but was ready to try again. It was touch and go with parasites and digestive issues, but I watched my diet carefully and the trip worked out well. I traveled to Glastonbury, England, in the summer of 2009.

Gallbladder Scare

In the fall of 2009, I started having what I thought were digestive problems. I would feel nauseous immediately after eating. It turned out to be gallbladder issues. I may have overworked it with all the liver flushes, but I was also getting healthier. It was a scare, though. When it comes to gallbladder issues, the only treatment doctors recommend is to remove the gallbladder. I have never been ready to voluntarily give up a body part, and eight years into my recovery, I wasn't ready to start.

2010 - RETURN OF LYME DISEASE SYMPTOMS

In mid-2010, I started getting Lyme disease symptoms again. This was alarming, as it had been five years since I stopped taking medication for Lyme and I was starting to get some of my life back. The practitioner I was seeing, Caren Coe in Austin, used a bioresonance machine, called the Asyra, which was exceptionally good at detecting Lyme disease and coinfections. The machine could also tell how old an infection was and what the energetic level of the infection was. This was very helpful, because in my case it indicated that these symptoms were due to old infections and the energetic level was much higher than a normal active physical infection. An active physical infection would show a low energetic level; however, on the machine my symptoms were showing an energetic level so high that it was no longer at the physical level. This indicated the symptoms were not really a return of the actual disease, but most likely a deeper layer of energy and bacteria being flushed out of my cells as the healing process went deeper into my body. That was a huge relief, though my faith in that machine was tested again and again over the coming months as more symptoms kept coming up. In the end, the machine was correct. It was a deeper level of healing and not a return of the illness. Without the proper testing tool, I would not have known that, and it would have sent me off the deep end emotionally thinking that the disease had returned.

2011 - The Move to Emotional Healing

Up until mid-2011, my attempts at resolving my chronic illness were strictly in the realm of physical healing. That was ten full years, but by late 2011, my physical healing had hit a wall. I could not move forward on any of my digestive issues, and there was no relief in sight. I have often come across the right practitioner at the right time who could help with what I was going through, but nothing was helping at that time. I had been hearing and reading about how emotional issues are the underlying cause of physical illness, and people had been telling me about emotional healing for quite some time. I rarely felt good emotionally, so in an effort to bring about further healing of my illness, I started the process of emotional healing. This process is discussed fully in "Part II - Emotional Healing" of this book. My physical healing efforts continued while I pursued emotional healing.

2012 - Gut Dysfunction

The visits to practitioners and the treatments continued, as always. Digestive issues stood out. I started researching gut dysfunction and gut flora in 2012. A doctor named Rey Ximenes, MD did a series of tests on my intestinal function. The tests showed I had an ample amount of gut flora in my intestines, but that the variety of the different strains of gut flora bacteria was not adequate. I read the book *Gut and Psychology Syndrome*, by Natasha Campbell-McBride, MD, and I learned how to make bone broth, which is one of the most healing foods for the gut. I learned how to cook healthy, organic meals. I did all I could, but there was still no progress in the digestive area. Still, life was better than it had been in previous years.

PARASITES RE-EMERGE WITH A VENGEANCE

In mid-2012 I saw that a trip to Egypt was available. I wanted to go, but wondered if my gut health was up to it, especially in regard to traveling to Egypt. In the fall I had a horrific parasite episode which overwhelmed my body. I had to resort to the ozonated olive oil, and that was equally difficult on my body. This put any travel in danger. I considered ozone insufflation, which I had heard of but never tried. It involves pumping ozone gas directly into the body through an orifice. The ozone then travels through the body tissues to reach a large portion of the body. I found a doctor in Austin, Ted Edwards, MD who does this, and tried it. Not much seemed to happen. I was feeling better though, either due to the treatment or just because the parasite episode had passed. I decided to go on the Egypt trip. It had been a long time between bad parasite episodes, so perhaps another one was way off in the future.

TRAVEL WITH PARASITES

However, a month later on the flight to Egypt, another parasite episode began. I had packed some ozonated olive oil and capsules just in case. I created a new way to get the gel into capsules without melting it, and I decided to take them every other day. The dose and frequency of treatment that might help me, without incapacitating me, were a total guess. I had never used this method, and the amount per capsule was difficult to calibrate. With ozonated olive oil, if you take too much you will be in pain and unable to move, and if you take too little it won't help. And in either case, you'd better be near a bathroom for about four hours after you take it to accommodate horrific diarrhea. Somehow, I got it just right. I took the right number of capsules every other evening. Then I would be fine for traveling on the bus the next day. It was a miracle to improvise that treatment and get all that right so that it did not interfere with the trip at all.

2013 - CHELATION OF HEAVY METALS & BLOOD TREATMENTS

HEAVY METAL CHELATION

The doctor I went to for ozone insufflation, Dr. Ted Edwards in Austin, also did heavy metal chelation, so I got tested to see what my metal levels were. They were high, so I started chelation of heavy metals in early 2013. Chelation treatments were ninety-minute sessions of an intravenous drip of EDTA, a solution which pulls heavy metals out of the body and eliminates them through the urinary tract. I did these twice per week. I continued that for thirty treatments and then tested again. While the levels of most metals had gone down, others had come up, which happens because when you clear out a layer of issues, the next layer emerges. I continued for another twenty treatments and stopped.

ULTRAVIOLET BLOOD TREATMENTS

Around this time, Dr. Edwards began doing ultraviolet blood treatments—blood was removed intravenously and run through a machine where ultraviolet light would kill pathogens before the blood was infused back into the body. I didn't know if it would help, so I tried it. It did help. I didn't know why at the time, though. It turned out that it was actually helping with a blood parasite that I had, though at the time I did not know that I had a blood parasite.

In the summer of 2013, I heard of a medical doctor from Trinidad who was visiting the country and giving sessions, Dr. Harry Ramnarine. He is an intuitive practitioner who uses numerical grids as part of his energy medicine practice. I decided to try a session. He diagnosed my biggest health issue as a blood parasite, and found the cause to be a lack of phosphorous in my blood. He tested to see which type of phosphorus would be best for my body, and found that a homeopathic treatment of phosphorous was the best way to restore my blood levels of phosphorous. It worked, and the parasite that had caused the terrible outbreak before the Egypt trip was now eliminated. Of course I still had many other types of parasites remaining, but the worst one was gone.

2013 - INTESTINAL INFECTION

Life was slowly improving through the first half of 2013, but in the summer, I developed a sharp, intermittent, shooting pain in my intestines, and discovered it was an intestinal infection. I didn't realize the consequences of this

at first. I did what I usually do. I went to health practitioners and medical intuitives, but the infection didn't go away.
After a few months of this, while researching, I realized
what was happening. I had done so much damage to my gut
flora (beneficial bacteria in the intestines) with antibiotic
treatments for Lyme, ten years earlier, that it could no
longer hold harmful bacteria in check. There was no good
way to kill this infection. Inside the intestines, the infection
is not connected to tissue with blood vessels, so antibiotics
could not get to it. Plus antibiotics are what caused the
problem in the first place by wiping out all the gut flora
which prevent this type of infection. The testing from 2012
had revealed that while I had an ample amount of gut flora
bacteria, I did not have the variety of strains of bacteria that
healthy gut flora contain.

DEAD END FOR GUT RECOVERY

This meant that there was no way to recover the gut flora I had lost due to long-term antibiotic use. I had been taking large amounts of probiotics for years, but that only
provides dozens of strains of good bacteria compared to the
over 500 strains of beneficial bacteria we have naturally in
our gut flora. So my twelve-year recovery back to health had
hit a brick wall, and had quite possibly reached checkmate. I
thought, *There's no way I could have come this far on this path
only to be stopped at this point.*

Intestinal infections can be debilitating and eventually
lead to being bedridden. Many people who have been bedridden for years with these infections eventually die. I was

six days away from a three-week trip to France when I realized all this. After twelve years of a great recovery from Lyme disease and chronic illness, was I now on the slow debilitating path to death? If I were to go on the trip and have problems, I might be put into a hospital where they would administer antibiotics. That would only make the problem worse.

MIRACLE SOLUTION EMERGES

As I frantically researched this issue, with pressure building only days before the trip, I quickly discovered the concept of the fecal transplant. I could not replace the gut flora I had lost, but I could acquire someone else's gut flora. There are online websites that describe this process and the issues involved. The difficult part is finding a healthy donor. First of all, do you really want to ask someone to do that? You need someone who has a healthy, regular digestive function, as you will acquire their digestive abilities. Then you have to make sure they have no infections or parasites that you would acquire through the transplant. Typically that would require testing, which would take a few weeks and cost over $1,000, but I had only six days before my trip. I was very lucky to find a donor who was knowledgeable enough about the body that no tests were needed. I performed the twenty-minute procedure and the problem was solved. I went on the trip to France for three weeks with no problems, and have never had a problem with intestinal infections again. Catastrophe avoided, recovery from chronic Lyme disease back on track.

2014 - DENTAL PROBLEMS

I've been told by intuitives that we store many of our unresolved emotional issues in our teeth—it is the only structure in the body that can handle them. Chapter 4 has charts that show the relationship between the emotions and teeth.

By 2014, I had been doing emotional healing for about two-and-a-half years (see "Part II - Emotional Healing"), and my teeth were acting up. I had lost one tooth in 2011. If you do not resolve the emotional issues stored in a tooth in time, you will not be able to save the tooth. It will have to be removed in order for the body to let go of the emotional issues stored in that tooth.

CAVITATION

I had pain in some of my teeth, and it was not clear what the problem was. As always, I had to resort to a combination of unusual means to figure this out. The bioresonance machine that my naturopath uses can do a teeth scan. It called out a cavitation on an upper front tooth. My chiropractor, John Bandy DC of Austin, is an expert at determining infections in teeth. He can find them long before a dentist can. He determined there was a cavitation between the roots of my two upper front teeth in the summer of 2014. Cavitations are pockets of infection in the jaw bone. Conventional dentistry typically doesn't acknowledge that cavitations even exist. Biological dentists do. When I had my root canals taken out in 2005, I was tested and found to have some cavitations. When the dentist drilled into the pockets of infection, I saw the white pus that he scooped out of them. They do exist, but typically cavitations occur after a tooth has been pulled, where the area may not have been cleaned properly. In my case in 2014, I had a cavitation between the roots of two live teeth, which is unusual. An expert with X-rays could possibly see it, but it was barely visible. I needed a dentist who used kinesiology to confirm the presence of infection. Even then, what can you do about it? Some dentists might drill into the jaw, but the likelihood of damaging the nerves of healthy teeth is high. I went to the dentist in Dallas who had done my work in 2005. He had a method of drilling through the gums into the pocket of infection and then injecting a homeopathic concoction into the pocket with a needle. The pain in the tooth cleared, but the infection was not quite healed. The cavitation caused more problems in late August a week before I was to travel to Bosnia (I seem to have a repeating pattern of having health crises before overseas trips). Another trip to Dallas with the homeopathic treatment, and the infection was completely healed.

JAW MISALIGNMENT

At this time I found that my lower and upper front teeth were bumping and causing pain. I had been working to adjust my posture, and it was misaligning my lower jaw. Braces were considered, but braces will lock a skull-to-spine-to-jaw alignment into your body. It was advised to resolve the posture issue before considering braces, and that the posture issue would most likely resolve the jaw misalignment.

Holding a lot of stress in the jaw can also cause it to go out of alignment.

This section on dental problems ties in more with "Part II - Emotional Healing" than with Lyme disease, though it illustrates that all levels of healing are interrelated.

2015 - Healing

My health issues reached a plateau again for a couple of years after 2013. I've learned to stop worrying about it and just live with it. Plus, I have been pretty healthy in the last two years, so this hasn't been difficult. In early 2015, after three full years of intensive work on emotional healing, I came across a spiritual teacher who taught a great deal about the concept of nonresistance. This concept is discussed in "Part III - Spiritual Healing" of this book. In the meantime, of course, my physical healing efforts continued, but they were mostly just maintenance efforts.

Chronic Illness Recovery Process

Recovery from chronic illness is not a linearly increasing process by which you get better little by little. Health seems to improve in quantum jumps, after which it reaches a plateau and stays about the same for quite some time, while the body consolidates its gains. In the meantime there are many crises and setbacks, and you might not feel good at all at times. In chronic illness, when many body systems are affected, you not only have to kill pathogens and detoxify the body, but then you have to bring the body systems back into balance with each other. As you keep healing, the whole system keeps changing, and it is a challenge to maintain balance. When you heal one level of issues and bring things into balance, a deeper level of issues emerges, throwing things out of balance again. It can look like you are losing ground in the healing process, but that's not the case. Sometimes there are even actual healing crises, like when you kill many pathogens at once and you overload the elimination systems, causing you to feel bad. Such a "crisis" can seem like a problem, when in fact your healing is breaking through to a higher level. Healing is a messy process which is difficult to measure according to how you feel.

New Nutritionist

In the summer of 2015, someone told me about a nutritionist in Austin named Joseph Strickland, who uses Nutrition Response Testing. I've discovered over time that when I wait patiently, I receive guidance on my healing path—I've often come across the right practitioner at just the right time. I've discovered that one way to receive this guidance is through serendipity, so when I got this recommendation out of the blue, I suspected it was time for another quantum leap in my health. I went to see Joe Strickland, and his work was a perfect fit for what I needed. My remaining issues were parasites, fungus, some remaining mercury, and my nervous system that was frozen. He was able to test my nervous system with a computer program which measures the autonomic nervous system based on heart rate variability. This program measures the parasympathetic nervous system while you are lying down and then the sympathetic nervous system while you are standing.

The autonomic nervous system consists of two branches—the sympathetic and the parasympathetic. The sympathetic nervous system activates to respond to stressful situations. It puts the body in fight-or-flight mode. The parasympathetic nervous system activates to calm the body and rest. It puts the body in relaxation and healing mode.

My parasympathetic nervous system has had trouble turning on throughout my whole life, after a birth trauma. This prevents the body from relaxing and going into healing mode. Joe found that my body's lack of enzyme production was interfering with the nervous system. When we addressed that through supplementation, my parasympathetic nervous system started to respond and switch on. That, in itself, will move the body's healing forward. I had been told for years that my parasympathetic nervous system was not shifting on properly, but no one could test it or resolve it. Joe also tested my levels of heavy metals. The only one that appeared was mercury. The mercury levels were not high, so more intravenous chelation was not needed. He decided to address the mercury through supplementation with the herbal supplement, Spanish Black Radish by Standard Process. He was able to measure the progress of mercury detoxification every week, and by the end of 2015 the mercury level was down about 75 percent from where we started. Parasites were still around, and we had to spend several months treating them; however, they were now finally leaving for good. Joe was able to test which parasites to treat and in which order. I would treat for ten days on herbs followed by five days off. Through testing, he found that we needed to treat parasites before getting more aggressive with fungus. I have found Joe Strickland to be one of the most skillful practitioners I've come across in the testing and treatment of parasites, as well as other chronic health issues.

2016 - Full Recovery

As of January 1, 2016, I am on my last ten-day round of parasite treatment. Then we will move on to the final step of cleaning up some minor fungus issues. This is now a full recovery.

There are no words for what it means to me to be parasite free. Looking back on it all now, this is a miracle. I know that I won a few battles with this illness, but it never felt like that. To summarize how this illness *felt* to me, I would say,

> *I felt like I lost every single battle that I ever fought against this huge, seemingly invincible illness for fourteen years. And then one day I woke up and discovered that I had won the war.*

[3]

General Outline of Chronic Lyme Treatment

GENERAL OUTLINE OF TREATMENT

- A way is needed to test for all the issues you have. A Lyme infection typically comes with coinfections like Ehrlichia, Babesia, and Bartonella. However, with chronic Lyme disease you also have fungi, viruses, toxins, allergies, and parasites.

- Once you can determine all the issues you have, you need a way to treat them all one-by-one. It's like peeling the layers of an onion: you treat the layer of issues presenting itself at present. Once you resolve the issues from that layer, the next layer of issues comes up, and you deal with those issues. You keep working with layer after layer until you are done.

- As you make your way through this process, it is helpful to have an objective way to measure your progress. You typically won't feel any better when you resolve issues because you have so many. It can be very discouraging to go year after year without feeling better, so a way to measure progress, aside from how you feel, is important. The testing methods will help.

- There are two routes of treatment: conventional medicine and alternative medicine:

  - Conventional medicine will typically only test for and treat Lyme disease and coinfections, and they are treated with antibiotics. Conventional medicine is covered by insurance.

  - Alternative medicine will test for and treat everything, and illnesses are treated with natural medications. Alternative medicine uses many testing methods: bioresonance or electrodermal machines, kinesiology, medical intuitives, and many others. No one practitioner will offer everything you need. Alternative medicine is typically not covered by insurance.

[4]

Discussion of Issues and Treatment Modalities

BREASTFEEDING & GUT FLORA

It is important to note that you may have had a long-standing problem with gut flora that preceded your illness and antibiotic use. According to Dr. Natasha Campbell-McBride in her book, *Gut and Psychology Syndrome*, babies who are breastfed develop completely different gut flora than babies who are bottle-fed. Babies are born with a sterile gut, so breastfeeding is essential to properly seed a baby's gut flora with the right mix of healthy bacteria (from the mother). In fact, breastfeeding is the only opportunity in our lives to develop the gut flora properly. Babies who are bottle-fed are seeded with a different mixture of bacteria, and are later prone to many health issues. A whole generation of people who were born in the 1960s and 1970s were not breastfed because it was out of fashion, and this has caused numerous health issues for that generation.[1]

GENERATIONAL EFFECT OF GUT FLORA DAMAGE

Dr. Campbell-McBride states that other factors which affect gut flora are birth control pills, antibiotics and poor diet. So not only do we have women who did not breastfeed in the 1960s and 1970s which compromised their gut flora. Then they passed on their compromised gut flora to their daughters, who consequently used birth control pills and degraded their flora further. The daughters then had their own children, and passed on their weak flora to them. It is easy to see a chain of events that could seriously degrade the gut flora of a significant portion of the population within two to three generations.

If you add to this process typical rounds of antibiotics in people's lives, and a poor diet including sugary foods and breakfast cereals for children, it is easy to see how we have a large portion of the population today with a compromised gut and immune problems.[2] And, of course, people with a compromised gut and immune problems acquire more infections requiring antibiotics, which further degrade their gut flora, which they then pass on to their children.

ANTIBIOTIC USE IN LYME DISEASE TREATMENT

Antibiotics are the first line of treatment against Lyme disease in conventional medicine, and conventional medicine is where most people start in their treatment of Lyme. As stated earlier, antibiotics work great in a case of acute

Lyme disease when treatment is started soon after infection and treatment is limited to a few weeks. However, antibiotics are not as effective against chronic Lyme disease which has been in the body for a longer period of time. This means antibiotics need to be taken for a much longer period of time which degrades the gut flora.

ANTIBIOTICS & GUT FLORA

Antibiotics are very effective at killing Lyme disease bacteria. Unfortunately, they also kill gut flora, which are the beneficial bacteria in your intestines. Gut flora are an integral part of the immune system, and they assist digestion and assimilation. If you take antibiotics for a short period of time, you can recover the gut flora through the use of probiotics. However, if you take antibiotics for an extended period of time, you risk harming the gut flora beyond repair, which can do permanent damage to your immune system. The worst case is when you are not able to get off the antibiotics, because the immune system is compromised. In this case you will get a test result that says there is no more Lyme, so you go off antibiotics, but the Lyme disease will quickly return because your immune system is not strong enough to take over after the antibiotics are discontinued. At this point you can never get off antibiotics.

The immune system is the best thing your body has going for it in regard to illness. It's wise not to harm it. Most people don't find this out until it's too late. This illness starts out with Lyme disease overwhelming the immune system. Then pathogens that the immune system normally holds in check are free to multiply. Antibiotics then damage the gut flora, which compromises the immune system. This facilitates Candida, other infections, and parasites. Mercury, dental toxins, fluoride, chlorine, and food additives also suppress the immune system, and the permanent loss of gut flora may mean no end to antibiotics. This is the downward spiral to serious health problems.

HERBAL PROTOCOLS FOR LYME

Dr. Cowden has created protocols with the herbal medications Samento and Banderol, by Nutramedix, which are quite effective against Lyme bacteria but do not harm the gut flora. See the "Cowden Support Program" on www.nutramedix.com.[3] Also, see "Killing Protocols" on www.lymediseaseresource.com[4] for protocols by many doctors, including Dr. Cowden. It may be challenging to find doctors who provide a protocol for Lyme disease that uses medications that do not harm gut flora.

EFFECTS OF GUT FLORA DAMAGE

While it may be possible to win the battle against Lyme disease using antibiotics, you may lose the war if you destroy your gut flora and damage your immune system. It can literally threaten your life. There are over 500 strains of beneficial bacteria in gut flora. Probiotic products contain only dozens of known strains, so if you take probiotics, you cannot recover all the bacterial strains you need. Several years later, you may start to develop intestinal infections, typically Clostridium difficile (C-diff). These can be difficult to treat. As stated earlier, they are inside the intestines and not connected to blood vessels, which would allow antibiotics to get to them. But antibiotics are what caused the problem in the first place by wiping out all the gut flora, so they would just make the problem worse anyway. You may be able to get rid of the current infection with antibiotics, but it will make it more likely that another infection will follow which will be more resistant to treatment. People with these types of intestinal infections can have so many problems that they become bedridden and eventually die. Thousands die every year from C-diff infections. See the section "Fecal Transplants" for further discussion.

I acquired my first intestinal infection in the summer of 2013, about ten years after stopping antibiotic use in 2003. The infection was causing intermittent shooting pains across my abdomen, which would last about five seconds. In the intervening years, I had taken an extraordinary amount of probiotics. In fact, intestinal testing had shown that the quantity of my gut flora bacteria was quite good. However, the variety of strains of the bacteria in the gut flora was no longer there, and my body could not fight off the infection. After several weeks I finally realized that the infection was not going away because I no longer had the right gut flora bacterial strains, and there was no way my body could replace them. That is when I discovered the fecal transplant, which is a quick, easy, and cheap procedure that can be used to replace your gut flora with that of another person. One treatment resolved the problem for me almost immediately.

If you are taking antibiotics for Lyme, it is recommended that you take probiotics as well. There are ways to support your gut flora during antibiotic treatment that may help you through the process. This is discussed further in the section "Rebuilding the Gut Flora."

NOTE: Many of the chronic illness issues discussed in the following sections were caused because I did Lyme disease treatments which severely damaged my gut flora. In fact, after I overcame Lyme disease in late 2005, it took another ten years to overcome all the issues created due to the damaged gut flora, and recovery was not certain. If you can treat Lyme disease with medications that do not harm the gut flora, you can avoid many of the most serious chronic health issues common among chronic Lyme disease patients discussed in the following sections. It may not be easy to find doctors who treat Lyme disease with medications that don't harm gut flora, but if you can do it, you may save yourself many years of misery trying to recover from chronic health issues.

CANDIDA

The destruction of gut flora facilitates the growth of the fungus Candida Albicans. Candida exists in a yeast form in a healthy, balanced body. Its ratio to other bacteria in the intestines is one yeast cell to one million bacteria.[5] The yeast does not overgrow because there is no room. It is crowded out by other bacteria. However, when there is a large bacteria die-off in the intestines due to antibiotic treatments, room is then available for yeast overgrowth to occur while all the different types of bacteria race to grow back after antibiotics are discontinued. Candida then mutates into a fungal form and spreads. It can affect the body physically and mentally. It harms the intestinal walls, helps create leaky gut, and excretes toxins which are harmful to the body. Many Lyme disease patients who took antibiotics for a long period of time wind up with a severe case of Candida. If you have taken antibiotics once in your life, you have already upset the healthy ratio of yeast to bacteria. The more times you take antibiotics the worse the imbalance gets. Once this ratio is thrown out of balance, it can be difficult to restore it.

You can do a simple home Candida test. When you wake up in the morning, before you put anything into your mouth, work up some saliva and spit it into a clear glass of water. Within 1-3 minutes, look in the glass. If there are strings coming down from your saliva you have Candida.

CANDIDA SYMPTOMS

Women know Candida as a yeast infection, but anyone can get it. When it appears in the mouth it is called thrush. While symptoms appear in localized places, it is a system-wide infection throughout the body. People who have Candida feel terrible after eating sugar. They have an upset stomach, fatigue, irritability, and mental confusion.

CANDIDA TREATMENT

You must eliminate sugar from your diet, and also rice, bread and potatoes. There are many natural products which can treat Candida, but it's best to treat the entire digestive system rather than just one part. I found that a product called Yeast Control by World Health Mall was pretty good at treating Candida, plus it was effective against parasites as well. However, if you don't eliminate sugar from your diet, rebuild your gut flora, and address the other issues of the digestive system, it will be difficult to eliminate Candida.

LEAKY GUT & FOOD ALLERGIES

The mucous lining of the small intestine is a semi-permeable membrane. It allows nutrients to pass through and enter the bloodstream, but prevents unwanted toxins and undigested food from passing through as well. In chronic illness, a toxic environment erodes the lining of the intestines, causing it to become permeable. Now, toxins, microbes, and food particles that would not normally be permitted to enter the system leak into the bloodstream.[6] This facilitates Candida and parasitic infections in the intestines, making the problem worse. As toxins and food particles enter the bloodstream, the immune system attacks them. The body can then make antibodies against its own tissues in an autoimmune response where the body attacks itself. This is one of the causes of food allergies. In chronic illness, it is wise to often alternate treatments and foods that you eat, because the body will quickly become allergic to any substance that you take regularly when you have leaky gut.

Recovery from chronic illness requires cleaning up the intestinal tract, eliminating parasites and Candida, rebuilding your gut flora, and patching the holes in the walls of your intestine. Glutamine is a supplement helpful in healing the lining of the intestines.

Rebuilding the Gut Flora

If your gut flora has been damaged, then your immune system is compromised. You will not digest or assimilate food, vitamins, or minerals very well, so it is difficult for your body to get nutrition. It may be possible to rebuild the gut flora. This is typically done by taking probiotic supplements. These products contain strains of beneficial bacteria. Whether you can successfully reseed your gut flora depends on how much has been lost, for how long, and what you are using to rebuild it. Lab tests are available to check on the health of your gut bacteria.

There are over 500 strains of beneficial bacteria that comprise the gut flora in your body. All the strains of bacteria available in commercial probiotics add up to several dozen, so you can never recover all the lost strains if you have severely damaged your gut flora. Not all strains of beneficial bacteria are critically important, however.

The Work of Nigel Plummer, PhD

Significant work has been done in this area by Nigel Plummer, PhD. He has found four strains of bacteria which are the basic building blocks that anyone would need to reseed the gut flora if it has been damaged. This group of strains is called Lab4, and it was developed by Dr. Plummer and his colleagues. Several companies offer probiotics which contain the Lab4 strains of bacteria. HLC is one such popular brand. Based on his research, Dr. Plummer believes it is best to use human strains of gut flora bacteria rather than vegetable or yogurt strains. He also believes it is best to use the few critically beneficial strains, as opposed to just going for multiple strains. He recommends taking probiotics with food rather than on an empty stomach. The pH of an empty stomach is around 1.8 to 2.6, which is acidic enough to destroy a large portion of any probiotics taken. The pH of the stomach after eating is around 3.5 to 4.3. This level of acidity allows probiotics to survive digestion and land in the intestines, where they can take hold. As for taking probiotics during a regimen of antibiotics, Dr. Plummer recommends taking the probiotics daily, a few hours away from the antibiotics. The antibiotics will kill the probiotics every day; however, the probiotics, during their short life each day, will take up space that will help prevent fungus from spreading.[7]

Not everyone agrees on all these points in regard to probiotics. Practitioners typically recommend taking probiotics before bedtime, and eating fermented vegetables has been used by many cultures historically. It would be wise to test for which probiotic strains your body wants, and when to take them, using kinesiology.

PREBIOTICS

Something to consider when taking probiotics are prebiotics. Prebiotics are the food source for probiotics. A prebiotic is typically a food fiber that grows in plants. The most common prebiotics are inulin and oligofructose (FOS). These can be consumed as powders. Some probiotics contain prebiotics already in them. Some foods which contain prebiotics are chicory root, Jerusalem artichoke, dandelion greens, garlic and onions.

FERMENTED FOODS

Another typical way of reseeding the gut flora is to eat fermented foods. Eating a wide assortment of fermented vegetables can help rebuild the gut flora. They are typically being offered in health food stores now as sauerkraut, kimchi, and fermented beets. It is also possible to buy starter kits so that you can prepare your own mixture of fermented vegetables. Just one-quarter to one-half cup of fermented vegetables, eaten with one to three meals per day, is all it takes to supplement your gut flora. Many cultures have consumed these products historically for their health benefits. Yogurt has also been consumed historically, though commercial yogurts found in grocery stores are loaded with sugar.

FERMENTED DRINKS

There are also fermented drinks such as kombucha and kefir. Kombucha is a tea fermented by a bacteria and yeast culture which is filled with probiotics. Kefir is a cultured, enzyme-rich drink made from milk and filled with probiotics. These products may contain sugar, so if you have parasites or Candida, they may not be helpful.

Fecal Transplant

For those who cannot rebuild their gut flora any other way, there is a cheap and easy treatment which can replace your gut flora with the flora of another person. It is called a fecal transplant, which uses another person's fecal sample. The sample is prepared and inserted rectally into your colon. After insertion you lie on your side for ten minutes and it is done. The entire process is easy and takes about twenty minutes to perform. There are several online sites that go into great detail on this procedure, and many YouTube videos are available as well. The difficult part is finding a healthy donor with a good digestive system who will provide a stool sample, as you will acquire many of the digestive abilities of the donor's system. It is important to test this person for any diseases or parasites, as you do not want to acquire those during the process. Typical lab tests for this purpose can run over $1,000.

Success Rates for Fecal Transplants

According to anecdotal evidence, one fecal transplant procedure is all that is needed for a person to fully recover from an intestinal infection in about 90 percent of cases. In the rest of the cases, multiple procedures are used. Overall, the percentage success rate is in the high nineties for all people who have done this procedure. There are many cases of people who had been bedridden for years due to intestinal infections, and had even reached their deathbeds, who did this procedure and were able to completely recover rather quickly. That is the value of gut flora. In my case, one treatment eliminated the intestinal infection. My symptoms were gone almost immediately after treatment.

Fecal Transplants & the FDA

Some doctors and hospitals perform this procedure, but not many. The FDA has not been very clear about how it will regulate the procedure. There are valid concerns about screening a donor for disease before performing the procedure, but 15,000 people are dying per year from Clostridium difficile (C-diff) infections in the intestines. Typical treatment of these infections is with antibiotics, but antibiotics killing off the gut flora is what caused the problem in the first place. Every time you treat with antibiotics, you make it more likely that you will get the infection again, and less likely that treatment will be effective. In January 2013, the *New England Journal of Medicine* published the first rigorous, head-to-head study showing that fecal transplants were superior to antibiotics for the treatment of patients with recurring C-diff infections.[8]

Parasites

Parasites are a big issue with Lyme. They typically come in through food. If they can survive stomach acid, they lodge in the intestines first but can then migrate to other parts of the body. They consume the highest quality nutrients of the food you eat, leaving only the leftovers for you. They also consume a large amount of minerals. If you have parasites, you will typically find that you are depleted of minerals. Parasites can commandeer your moods and make you irritable. They can make you feel tense and cause anger episodes to erupt. Parasites lay a lot of eggs, so ongoing treatment is necessary as new waves of eggs hatch. The full moon is a typical time when parasites get really active and hatch a lot of eggs, and you will find that symptoms are magnified then. To resolve parasite issues, you will also need to work on your emotional issues (see "Part II - Emotional Healing" of this book).

Parasite Testing

To treat parasites, you will need a practitioner who can accurately test for them, test for which herbs to take for them, and test what order to treat them in. It is best to test often enough to monitor this process for modifications that may be needed when new parasites show up, or when the herbs become ineffective. Conventional medicine testing for parasites can be tricky. Stool samples are typically used, but even intestinal parasites don't show up in stool samples all the time, so a good test would need to be done over several days. Not all parasites reside in the intestines though. They can burrow into your abdominal organs and go elsewhere in the body. In this case they would not show up in a stool test at all. In alternative medicine, kinesiology is effective for parasite testing. Bioresonance testing machines are quite good, and medical intuitives can be good also. I never relied on any one type of test or treatment. Each type of test gives a look at the situation from a different viewpoint. Various types of tests can be used to verify each other.

PARASITE TREATMENT INTERVALS

While ongoing treatment is needed, it is important to take brief breaks. Parasite eggs will not hatch in an environment where they will immediately die, as is the case during treatment, so short breaks in treatment encourage the eggs to hatch. The resumption of treatment then proceeds to kill the newly hatched parasite eggs. I have been using a treatment cycle of ten days on and five days off. It is pretty successful but sometimes needs modification. For large parasites I've had to go to ten days on and two days off. Parasites sometimes consume the eggs of other parasites. In my most recent parasite treatment, we were using the Bio Challenge Systemic Formulas—four herbal formulations for large, small, microscopic, and cellular parasites (VRM1 to VRM4). In this case testing showed that we were to start treating the smallest and move upward. We wiped out the cellular parasites first, then the microscopic, and then the small ones. Only the large ones remained. After a few rounds of treatment on the large parasites, the small ones suddenly appeared again. The large parasites had consumed the eggs of the small ones, and when the bodies of the large ones were killed and started decomposing, the eggs of the small ones spilled out and hatched. So we were back to treating two types. It was important to test every two weeks in order to stay on top of new developments.

Parasite Remedy Rotation

It is best to rotate parasite remedies, because the parasites mutate, which makes successive treatments ineffective. I have found natural remedies to be best. The little experience I had with pharmaceutical drugs for treating parasites was not very good. Either the drugs were ineffective, or they became ineffective quickly due to parasite mutations. The first time I used a drug, Albendazole, it wiped out the adult parasites completely, but two weeks later new eggs had hatched and grown. The next time I took Albendazole, it was only fifty percent as effective as the first time. Parasites are skilled at mutating into forms that are resistant to treatment.

Common Herbs for Parasite Treatment

The most common herbs used for parasite treatment are black walnut hulls, wormwood, and cloves. Other treatments include raw garlic, diatomaceous earth, oil of oregano, and pumpkin seeds. There are many other herbs used to treat parasites. It is best to use proprietary mixtures of herbs found in health food stores, preferably prescribed by a practitioner who can test for the best remedy for your body using kinesiology, or some other testing method.

Treatment for Ascaris Lumbricoides

As discussed earlier, Ascaris lumbricoides is a common roundworm parasite. I used the recommendations by Hulda Clark of the Dr. Clark Information Center and used ozonated olive oil.[9] My experience was that ozonated olive oil works like a nuclear weapon against roundworm. It wipes them all out. The parasites cannot mutate away from it. If you have a heavy Ascaris parasite load, start slowly. Ozonated olive oil can be made at home or bought online. It is a gel that needs to be kept refrigerated to stay in gel form and keep its effectiveness. The taste is truly horrific, so it is best not to take it straight. I would take the gel out of the refrigerator, put some in a small glass, put the glass in a pot of water, and heat it in order to melt it down to a liquid. Then I would use a dropper to put the liquid into capsules and freeze the capsules for later use. I have also used Hulda Clark's zapper on parasites. It had an effect, but did not wipe them all out. I had too many types of parasites for them to be wiped out with any one treatment.

PARASITES & VIRUSES

Parasites can carry viruses in their bodies, so when you kill them and their bodies decompose, the viruses in their bodies are released into your body. I often got viruses of this type. They would make me miserable for a week, until I realized what they were and how to treat them. I would start to feel an upset stomach shortly after eating. For years I thought the viruses were coming from my food because the virus was always triggered after eating. I discovered that I could take an antiviral herb for these viruses.

There are two herbal products from Nutramedix, Noni and Takuna, that can treat these viruses. The sooner I started treatment after feeling bad, the better. I would take a dropper of the herb in a little water every half hour until I felt better, and then take it less often after that until the discomfort was completely gone. It can take several hours to knock out a virus of this type. The longer you wait to start treatment, the longer it takes to wipe it out. If you wait too long, you won't be able to get it under control at all, and you will be sick for a week. Going to sleep can be a problem. If you go several hours without treatment while sleeping, the virus will gain a lot of strength, and by morning it may be too late to get it under control again.

STOMACH ACID

It is helpful to test your stomach's acid production. Stomach acid is the first line of defense against parasites that have been ingested with food. Medications for acid reflux in recent years have become popular, but they decrease stomach acid production, which can reduce your protection against parasites. Over time, they train your body to produce less acid, so it may be necessary to train your stomach to produce a normal amount of acid again. Acid reflux can be caused by too much or too little stomach acid, so it is best not to just arbitrarily take a medication that cuts your acid production. It might make the acid reflux worse, and it will reduce your parasite defenses.

LONG-TERM PARASITE TREATMENT

If you have a significant parasite infestation you will have to grind them down over time. And you have to get their eggs shortly after hatching. Some lay hundreds of thousands of eggs per day. If you are not on top of the situation it will get out of hand. This process took me 14 years, but I didn't always have the correct timing. Different practitioners do things differently. Find a practitioner who knows what he is doing in this regard. One of the most important things you can do with parasites is to deal with the emotional issues you have in regard to parasites. This is discussed in "Part II - Emotional Healing."

DENTAL ISSUES

AMALGAM FILLINGS

There is research showing that mercury in amalgam fillings leaches out of the teeth and lodges in your body tissues.[10] Every time you chew food, mercury vapor is released and gets absorbed by body tissue. Mercury can have a lot of adverse reactions on your health. In regard to Lyme bacteria, mercury can contribute to its resistance from antibiotic treatment. I found a good biological dentist and had my amalgam fillings replaced with a more suitable material. Drilling into the fillings can cause mercury vapors to be released, so there are procedures for amalgam filling removal that a biological dentist will use to capture the mercury vapor as well as the filling material. Otherwise, the process of amalgam filling removal itself would be a cause of mercury poisoning. There are several alternate filling materials which can be used. The dentist I was seeing used kinesiology to determine the best filling material for my body.

HEAVY METAL CHELATION

After removing the amalgam fillings with mercury, it is then necessary to do chelation treatments to remove the mercury (and other metals) from your body. Mercury has been leaching out of your fillings and into your body tissues since the day those fillings were put in. There are also many other metals in your body that harm your immune system which can be removed through chelation. Some of the more common ones that are tested for are: aluminum, arsenic, barium, bismuth, cadmium, cesium, lead, nickel, thallium, tin, and tungsten. Chemical chelation involves many sessions with an intravenous solution of EDTA (ethylene diamine tetra-acetic acid), a synthetic amino acid. EDTA binds to heavy metals and minerals in the blood, so that they can be excreted in the urine. A chelating session lasts for about ninety minutes. The cost per session when I did the treatments in 2013 was about $175 per treatment. I did fifty such treatments. The low level of mercury I have tested for recently is addressed through supplementation with Spanish Black Radish by Standard Process. It is important to be tested for the right dosage. You don't want to detoxify more mercury than your elimination systems can handle, or the mercury can get reabsorbed into your body. Chlorella has also been a well-known detoxifier of metals in the body; however, parasites like to eat chlorella. If you later do a parasite cleanse, it may release the mercury back into your system as the parasites die, so if you have used chlorella, you might want to test for mercury after you do a parasite cleanse.

Root Canal Toxicity

Another treatment which can be very helpful is to remove teeth that have root canals. Every tooth has several miles of microscopic tubules which contain living tissue. When the tooth root is removed during a root canal procedure, this effectively kills the tooth. The tooth remains in place, but it is dead. However, all the living tissue in the microscopic tubules of the tooth remains in place, because it cannot be cleaned out. This living tissue dies and produces toxins which drip into your body every day for the rest of your life. This is another toxic load that the immune system has to carry. If you have several root canals, this multiplies the toxic load. If your immune system is already overloaded, this additional toxic load can be very harmful. In a video, biological dentist Dr. Stuart Nunnally explains that he tests the root canalled teeth that he removes from patients, and has found evidence of some of the worst types of bacteria in these teeth.[11]

Replacing Lost Teeth

If you don't use root canals, then what do you do if you need to pull teeth? I have had one tooth pulled in recent years and just left the open gap because the tooth was not very visible. Removing teeth becomes a concern when the teeth are visible or your molars are needed for chewing.

Implants can be risky health-wise, according to alternative health practitioners. Titanium implants are not good because that metal does not transmit energy in the body. Conventional dentists do not concern themselves with energy considerations; however, alternative practitioners are very aware of how the energy systems in the body affect health. Some people with titanium implants have serious problems due to the blocked flow of energy in their jaw, and they need to have the expensive implants removed. There are now implants made of crystalline material which is a better solution, but there are still differences of opinion on that. In my case, I opt to not put any foreign materials in my body if at all possible. If I were to lose several molars, I would be tempted to consider crystalline implants.

Bridges can be used to replace missing teeth, but it is necessary to damage the two anchor teeth on either side of the pulled tooth. This can lead to an early loss of the anchor teeth. Keep in mind also that a bridge will put extra pressure on the anchor teeth. When chewing food, the same biting force that would have been distributed to three teeth originally, is now distributed only to two teeth, which is a 50% increase in pressure to each of the anchor teeth.

Partial dentures are one of the better alternatives. They are made of a type of plastic. They are removable and snap in. Pay attention to the material they are made of. The ones that are pink in color to match the gums have been found to have heavy metals in them such as cadmium. Clear plastic can be used which does not contain any metals.

DENTAL CARE

You can also take better care of your teeth. This idea starts to make sense after you lose a few teeth. I use an ionic toothbrush from Soladey which does not require toothpaste and is remarkable at removing tartar. At night I also brush my teeth with a hydrogen peroxide solution to neutralize any bacteria that would work on my teeth while I sleep. According to dentist Weston Price, the best way to care for your teeth is through a good diet of real food. Dr. Price studied the effect of diet on the dental health of indigenous cultures back in the 1930s. He also did interesting research on root canals. The Weston Price Foundation offers a lot of the research on diet that Dr. Price did.[12]

DENTAL CHART

When linking health issues with dental issues, it is good to refer to a dental chart which links the teeth to organs and emotional issues (see Figures 1a and 1b).[13] These items are all connected energetically through acupuncture meridians. The few teeth I have lost are linked to the body systems and emotions that I have had issues with.

For example, I lost tooth #4 in 2011 after starting emotional healing. As per Figure 1a, the emotional issues related to that tooth are chronic grief, over criticalness, sadness, and controlling behaviors. The related body parts are the sinus and also the large intestine. Well, the emotional issues are accurate. And at the time, I had a sinus infection that was difficult to get rid of which was affecting the root of the tooth, and my long-term parasite issues have been in the large intestine.

So if you are having a problem with a tooth, it is a good idea to look at this chart to see what the underlying causes might be.

Loneliness, Acute Grief, Humiliated, Trapped, Inhibited, Lack Joy Greed, Not lovable	Anxiety, Self-Punishment, Broken Power, Hate, Low self-worth, Obsessed	Chronic Grief, Overcritical, Sadness, Controlling, Feeling trapped, Dogmatic, Compulsive, Uptight	Anger, Resentment Frustration, Blaming, Incapable to take action, Manipulative	Fear, Shame, Guilt, Broken will, Shyness, Helpless, Deep exhaustion
Duodenum Middle Ear, Shoulder Elbow, CNS S-I joint, foot, toes	Sinus: Maxillary Oropharynx, Larynx	Sinus: Paranasal and Ethmoid, Bronchus, Nose	Sinus: Sphenoid Palatine Tonsil Hip, Eye, Knee	Sinus: Frontal Pharyngeal Tonsil Genito-Urinary System
	Right Breast			
Heart, Small Int., Circulation/Sex, Endocrine	Pancreas Stomach	Lung Large Intestine	Liver Gallbladder	Kidney Bladder

1	2	3	4	5	6	7	8
32	31	30	29	28	27	26	25

Heart, Small Int., Circulation/Sex, Endocrine	Lung Large Intestine	Pancreas Stomach	Liver Gallbladder	Kidney Bladder
Shoulder, Elbow Ileum, Middle Ear Peripheral Nerves S-I joint, foot, toes	Sinus: Paranasal and Ethmoid, Bronchus, Nose	Sinus: Maxillary Larynx, Lymph, Oropharynx / Right Breast	Sinus: Sphenoid Palatine Tonsil Hip, Eye Knee	Sinus: Frontal Ear, Pharyngeal Tonsil Genito-Urinary System
Loneliness, Acute Grief, Humiliated, Trapped, Inhibited, Lack Joy Greed, Not lovable	Chronic Grief, Overcritical, Sadness, Controlling, Feeling trapped, Dogmatic, Compulsive, Uptight	Anxiety, Self-Punishment, Broken Power, Hate, Low self-worth, Obsessed	Anger, Resentment Frustration, Blaming, Incapable to take action, Manipulative	Fear, Shame, Guilt, Broken will, Shyness, Helpless, Deep exhaustion

Figure 1a (right side of body)

Fear, Shame, Guilt, Broken will, Shyness, Helpless, Deep exhaustion	Anger, Resentment Frustration, Blaming, Incapable to take action, Manipulative	Chronic Grief, Overcritical, Sadness, Controlling, Feeling trapped, Dogmatic, Compulsive, Uptight	Anxiety, Self-Punishment, Broken Power, Hate, Low self-worth, Obsessed	Loneliness, Acute Grief, Humiliated, Trapped, Inhibited, Lack Joy Greed, Not lovable
Sinus: Frontal Pharyngeal Tonsil Genito-Urinary System	Sinus: Sphenoid Palatine Tonsil Hip, Eye, Knee	Sinus: Paranasal and Ethmoid, Bronchus, Nose	Sinus: Maxillary Oropharynx Larynx	Ileum, Jejunum Middle Ear, Shoulder Elbow, CNS S-I joint, foot, toes
		Left Breast		
Kidney Bladder	**Liver Gallbladder**	**Lung Large Intestine**	**Stomach Spleen**	**Heart, Small Int., Circulation/Sex, Endocrine**

9	10	11	12	13	14	15	16
24	23	22	21	20	19	18	17

Kidney Bladder	**Liver Gallbladder**	**Spleen Stomach**	**Lung Large Intestine**	**Heart, Small Int., Circulation/Sex, Endocrine**
Sinus: Frontal Ear, Pharyngeal Tonsil Genito-Urinary System	Sinus: Sphenoid Palatine Tonsil Hip, Eye Knee	Sinus: Maxillary Larynx, Lymph, Oropharynx Knee	Sinus: Paranasal and Ethmoid, Bronchus, Nose	Shoulder, Elbow Ileum, Jejunum, Middle Ear Peripheral Nerves S-I joint, foot, toes
		Left Breast		
Fear, Shame, Guilt, Broken will, Shyness, Helpless, Deep exhaustion	Anger, Resentment Frustration, Blaming, Incapable to take action, Manipulative	Anxiety, Self-Punishment, Broken Power, Hate, Low self-worth, Obsessed	Chronic Grief, Overcritical, Sadness, Controlling, Feeling trapped, Dogmatic, Compulsive, Uptight	Loneliness, Acute Grief, Humiliated, Trapped, Inhibited, Lack Joy Greed, Not lovable

Figure 1b (left side of body)

LIVER FLUSHES & GALLSTONES

Liver flushes are great for liver congestion in chronic illness. The liver filters out toxins and all kinds of material from your blood, and also performs other critical functions. In chronic illness, the liver can get overloaded and congested, which means it is clogged with hardened globs of bile. Doing liver flushes is one of the few procedures I ever did that made me feel better, at least for a couple of days after the flush. I started doing liver flushes because I found out I had gallstones in 2006, and I did not want to have surgery to remove my gallbladder. Gallstones are an issue that seems to come up often with Lyme disease and chronic illness. The procedures flushed out a lot of stones from my liver and gallbladder, however I found out that people with certain emotional issues will tend to keep creating stones, and I was one of those people. So I had to continue with flushes to keep cleaning out my system until such time as I resolved the emotional issues which kept me producing stones. I also learned from practitioners that a lot of anger issues are held in fat deposits in the liver, and liver flushes help to flush out this material as well. The effect of emotional issues on physical health are addressed in "Part II - Emotional Healing".

THE LIVER FLUSH PROCEDURE

My gallbladder has remained in good health. To date I've done seventy-nine liver flushes since 2006. The procedure I used can be found in the book *The Amazing Liver and Gallbladder Flush* by Andreas Moritz. The book is a short, easy read, and explains a great deal about liver function and the benefits of doing liver flushes, as well as a step-by-step procedure for doing the actual flush. The flush process involves softening the stones for six days by drinking apple juice, and then drinking a combination of olive oil and grapefruit juice on the night of the flush just before going to bed.[14] The next day you will release many stones in several bowel movements throughout the morning. The bowel movements consist of only water and stones.

Gallstones

Stones in this case refer to the hardened globs of bile which get caught in the liver and gallbladder. These are typically soft and green in color. It is also possible that a few stones that have been around a long time will have hardened and calcified, but these are rare. These will turn white in color and can be found on an X-ray.

Softening Stones

Note that if you have parasites or Candida, you cannot be drinking large amounts of apple juice to soften the stones due to the sugar content. One alternative is to take malic acid powder in water. Malic acid is the part of apple juice that softens the stones. There are other herbs to soften stones as well. At times I have used orthophosphoric acid combined with the herb Hydrangea. Another option is gold coin grass, an herb used in traditional Chinese medicine. There is also the herb chanca piedra, from the Amazon rainforest, which is used to make tea that will help break down stones.

STONES & BILE DUCTS

As the diameter of the flushed stones is often bigger than the diameter of the tubes they flow through (common bile duct and cystic duct from the gallbladder), it is wise to take precautions. The process in the book involves drinking a series of glasses of Epsom salts in water before the flush, which has the effect of dilating the bile ducts so that the stones can move through more easily. A good website on liver flushes is www.sensiblehealth.com. It recommends two other products from traditional Chinese medicine. These are the herbal liquids curcumin and coptis, and they help lubricate the ducts so that the stones will pass through more easily.[15]

I have routinely passed stones up to 20 mm in diameter through bile ducts, which have an average 4 mm diameter, with no discomfort. I only experienced pain one time during one of my seventy-nine liver flushes. That was for fifteen minutes during one flush when I could feel a stone move through the cystic duct (duct from the gallbladder to the common bile duct) after coming out of my gallbladder. The pain was moderate. Practitioners who work with people doing liver flushes have told me of only a few cases when a person experienced discomfort during a flush.

DIET & GALLSTONES

When you have gallstones, foods that can irritate the gallbladder are meats high in fat, fried foods, acidic foods, dairy products, and refined foods. Coffee and chocolate are irritants as well. When I first found out I had gallstones, I immediately switched to a vegetarian diet to stop irritating my gallbladder (because of the stones). Years later, I came to the conclusion that it was best to keep the gallbladder working in order to keep the bile flowing, so I switched back to eating meat. My gallbladder was much healthier at that point. Different sources say that two to three week intervals are good for doing liver flushes. In the beginning you are anxious to improve your health, but after a while it is good to slow down. This is a significant procedure for the liver.

TRADITIONAL CHINESE MEDICINE ORGAN CLOCK

It is good to note the traditional Chinese medicine (TCM) organ clock that shows the time of day when each organ is functioning optimally and has the most energy. There are twelve organs, each having a two-hour increment on the twenty-four hour clock. During the two-hour interval for each organ, the energy flow through that organ is stimulated. It is the body's maintenance schedule for the organs. The gallbladder is affected from 11 p.m. to 1 a.m., and the liver is affected from 1 a.m. to 3 a.m. When I was having problems with my liver and gallbladder, it was causing insomnia usually between 1 a.m. and 3 a.m. If you have insomnia at a regular hour of the night, it is useful to check the organ chart to see which organ might be affected. The TCM organ clock is as follows.

ORGAN	**TIME PERIOD**
Lung	3 - 5 a.m.
Large Intestine	5 - 7 a.m.
Stomach	7 - 9 a.m.
Spleen	9 - 11 a.m.
Heart	11 a.m. - 1 p.m.
Small Intestine	1 - 3 p.m.
Urinary Bladder	3 - 5 p.m.
Kidney	5 - 7 p.m.
Pericardium	7 - 9 p.m.
Triple Burner	9 - 11 p.m.
Gallbladder	11 p.m. - 1 a.m.
Liver	1 - 3 a.m.[16]

GALLBLADDER SURGERY VERSUS LIVER FLUSHES

You must do your own due diligence and research before deciding a course of action. There are potential risks to liver flushes. Theoretically, stones can get stuck. There are also potential risks to gallbladder surgery. If a surgical instrument nicks a bile duct it can cause excruciating pain, and possibly more severe consequences depending on the damage and interval before treatment. Some people who have had their gallbladders removed do really well. Many do not. There can be some real limitations on eating fat.

A doctor once recommended not to remove any body parts unless my life was in danger. I have found this to be good advice. I know of too many people who have had surgery to remove gallbladders (and other parts) who found out later that there were other options. The problem is that you cannot put a body part back in after you take it out.

DIET

Diet is a huge issue in chronic illness. Food is the main source of nutrition for your body. It is wise to eat organic foods. Processed foods have too many harmful additives and are barely food at all. Research is showing more and more that GMOs are harmful to health. Even if GMOs themselves were safe, they were developed so that high doses of pesticides could be sprayed on them to get a good harvest. So pesticide doses are now many times higher than they used to be. Much of this washes off into our drinking water. Farm animals and poultry are routinely given antibiotics, so meat, milk, and eggs will provide us with antibiotic residues which damage our gut flora.

FISH

There aren't many good options left with fish. Some types have mercury contamination. The worst offenders are tuna, sea bass, marlin, and halibut. Farmed fish are not a healthy option. Wild Alaskan salmon is one of the few remaining good choices.

GRAINS

Whole grains are considered best, but some people believe grains are not healthy at all, like Dr. Joseph Mercola,

DO, who has authored many articles on the subject on his website and in his newsletters.[17]

SUGAR & SWEETENERS

Sugar is not good for a chronic illness patient. Anyone with parasites or Candida knows that eating sugar will cause great discomfort because parasites and Candida both love to consume sugar. Even if there is no discomfort, sugar inhibits the immune system. It slows down the reaction of white blood cells, which are the main defense against pathogens. Sugar negatively impacts the body in other ways as well. If you are serious about recovering from chronic illness, elimination of sugar from the diet is a necessity. Artificial sweeteners are not good either. Aspartame accounts for over 75 percent of all adverse food reactions reported to the FDA, and some are quite serious. The scientists who discovered Splenda were trying to create new insecticides by combining chlorine compounds with sugar, when they accidentally discovered that one had a sweet taste. According to the book *Sweet Deception*, by Joseph Mercola, DO, testing on artificial sweeteners was woefully inadequate before the FDA allowed these products on the market with sweeping safety claims that were unfounded.[18] Stevia is a possible alternative for a sweetener. It is an herb which has been used in Japan for decades. Taste varies between brands. I have found the Stevita brand to be a reasonable alternative to sugar. Cutting sugar out of a diet is a big job. Sugar is in so many things as high-fructose corn syrup, or just corn syrup, so you have to look at labels all the time. When I first attempted to eliminate sugar from my diet, it was also necessary for me to cut out bread, rice, and potatoes, as these items digest into forms of sugar which feed Candida and parasites. It took me a few years to become completely free of the sugar addiction.

JUICING

Fruit juice is not a good option, as the fiber in the fruit that regulates the body's absorption of sugar is stripped out in the juicing process. This will cause a blood sugar spike in your body when you drink the juice. Vegetable juice is a good option, though it is labor intensive. For those that are time challenged, green powder drinks can be a good way to add nutrients quickly and easily.

SALADS

Avocados are loaded with nutrients. An organic salad with sprouts, olives, nuts, some avocado and vegetables is a quick, easy, healthy meal. Shiitake mushroom salad dressing has no sugar and tastes good. Braggs' Liquid Aminos is a good liquid product that can be added to a salad to get a dose of amino acids.

PROTEIN SHAKES

For breakfast a protein shake with chocolate protein powder, avocado, coconut oil, wheatgrass powder, aloe vera juice, and sweetened with Stevia is healthy and tastes good.

Fermented Foods & Drinks

As mentioned in the section "Rebuilding Gut Flora", it is wise to eat fermented vegetables such as sauerkraut or kimchi. Just one-quarter to one-half cup of fermented vegetables, eaten with one to three meals per day, offers a large amount of good bacteria to fortify the gut flora, and could dramatically benefit your health. These can be purchased in health food stores or made at home with a starter kit.

Fermented drinks such as kombucha and kefir can also be helpful, though they may contain sugar.

Minerals & Enzymes

Sea salt or Pink Himalayan salt are good options for salt, as they contain many minerals. I found it was a good idea to take digestive enzymes with meals, because my body was not producing enough enzymes to digest food properly during my illness.

Diet Types

So what is the best diet? Paleo, vegetarian, vegan, raw food, nutritional typing, blood type, Hippocrates, yeast, the Maker's diet? The answer is no one knows. All have their good points and not so good points. Different things resonate with different people. It's best to listen to your body and eat what makes your body feel good. Experiment with different diets. Eat real food, which is food that is in the same form in which it came in nature. Find foods that taste good. Joy in life is important, and the joy of eating is part of that. Eat foods that you like. If your diet makes life miserable, it defeats the purpose of healing . . . and living.

At one point or another, I tried all of the above-mentioned diets and more. They were interesting and all had their good points, though none were fun. With so many differing viewpoints, it is necessary to read many books, experiment with many diets, and use your own wisdom to decide.

FILTERED WATER

Tap water has a lot of contaminants. Chlorine is harmful to the immune system. It is another load on the immune system while it is trying to battle chronic illness. Fluoride is another contaminant which is added to the drinking water in most cities. Many studies nowadays are showing it to be harmful to health. Even if fluoride were safe, it would be unwise to dose an entire population with it. Some people drink more water than others, and some have greater sensitivity to fluoride. If it were truly being used for better health, then the authorities would use pharmaceutical grade fluoride. However, they do not. Most sources of fluoride added to drinking water are industrial waste products. Studies also show that ingesting fluoride does not help tooth decay, which is the reason it was implemented in the first place. In fact, it does more harm than good.

To filter chlorine, I use a drinking water filter and a shower filter. The body absorbs chemicals through the skin as well as through ingestion, so both filters are helpful. Fluoride is not so easy to filter. Berkey has a fluoride filter for drinking water. There is no easy solution for fluoride in shower water. A reverse osmosis filter can filter all the water to a home, though it removes minerals from the water. In that case, it may be wise to add minerals back to the water before drinking it. This type of filter may not be an option for apartment living.

EXERCISE

The lymphatic system is part of the circulatory system. It is a network of lymph vessels that carries a clear fluid called lymph toward the heart. This fluid flows through the cells of the body, picking up waste materials which get filtered out by the lymph nodes. Unlike blood, this lymph fluid does not have a pump like the heart to move the fluid. The movement of lymph fluid is caused by body movement and breathing. So if you suffer from a chronic illness and your body is quite toxic, this system of waste disposal can be very important. Think of a town where the garbage has not been collected in many weeks. The garbage starts to pile up in the street and rot. If the lymphatic system is working overtime to rid the cells of waste, and the movement of the lymph fluid is not maintained, the body will back up with toxins and you won't feel well. Therefore, it is a good idea to maintain an exercise regimen, if only to keep the lymphatic system moving. Walking helps. If you are short on time for exercise, get a rebounder, which is a small trampoline. You can bounce on it several times a day. This will help keep your lymphatic fluids moving.

CLEANSES

Herbal cleanses are useful for detoxifying the body. You can buy these in a health food store, or have a practitioner design one and monitor it for you. There is an order in which to do cleanses. For instance, it is important to cleanse the colon before cleansing major organs. It may also be necessary to clear parasites out before doing an organ cleanse, as parasites can interfere with the results. You want to have your elimination channels clear so that when you flush out harmful toxins from your organs, they can be eliminated properly.

HYDROTHERAPY

The colon becomes backed up and extremely toxic in those with a chronic illness due to parasites, Candida, and other issues. As your body becomes toxic, all elimination channels can get backed up. Parasites create a mucous layer under which they can live their lives siphoning off critical nutrients from your diet for their own benefit. Colon hydrotherapy treatments, or colonics, are a way to flush your colon with water and hopefully get things moving again. An enema does not use enough water for this purpose. An analogy of the effect of using an enema to clean your colon (as opposed to a colonic), would be like trying to wash your car with a glass of water. An enema only flushes the last six inches of the colon, whereas a colonic uses enough water to flush the entire colon.

There are colon hydrotherapy treatment practitioners that you can see to perform a colonic. They are usually knowledgeable about fasting cleanses, which can be helpful to your health. There are also home colonic kits available online so that you can do this yourself. Colonics are good with liver flushes to make sure that flushed stones don't get caught in the intestines, where they may cause discomfort.

SAUNAS & STEAM BATHS

The skin is the largest organ in the body. It eliminates waste in the form of perspiration. Heat causes the lymphatic fluid to release toxins in the form of sweat. Anything that causes you to sweat can be helpful in releasing toxins from the body. However, raising the core temperature of the body, as in saunas and steam baths, has its own beneficial effects on the immune system. Infrared saunas have become popular with practitioners—they use lower temperatures, the heat penetrates the body more deeply, and they produce more sweat.

If you don't have access to a sauna or steam bath, it is helpful to just take a hot bath in your home. You can add herbs and essential oils to the bath for help with detoxification. There are also commercially available products in health food stores to add to a bath to help with detoxification.

Skin brushing is something you can do before bathing to increase lymphatic flow and detoxification. You take a brush and lightly brush your skin in the direction of your heart. This will stimulate the flow of lymphatic fluid as it carries toxins to the lymph nodes to be eliminated.

IONIC FOOTBATHS

Ionic foot baths have become popular. They have an element that creates ions that pull toxins out of your body through your feet. I used one many times. It was recommended by my doctor, but I don't know exactly what his criteria were for determining its effectiveness. I was not able to verify how well it worked.

OZONE INSUFFLATION

Ozone is a form of oxygen, O^3. It can be deadly to pathogens in the body. As mentioned earlier, ingesting ozonated olive oil can be deadly to certain types of parasites. Insufflation is another way of getting ozone to the interior of the body by inserting a tube into a body orifice and pumping in ozone gas. Not many doctors will perform this procedure. I found one and tried it for parasites using rectal insufflation into the large intestine. At the time, the parasite I was trying to dispatch was a blood parasite, but I did not know that. I thought it was an intestinal parasite, so the insufflation into the large intestine was not really effective at that time. I have no other experience with this procedure.

CARPAL TUNNEL SYNDROME

Carpal tunnel syndrome is another issue that seems to pop up with Lyme disease and chronic illness. I acquired it early on in my illness. It got progressively worse to the point where I had to wear temporary casts on both my wrists to alleviate the pain. The doctor recommended surgery, but I found a book called *Overcoming Repetitive Motion Injuries the Rossiter Way*, by Rossiter and MacDonald, that recommended exercises to eliminate carpal tunnel syndrome.[19] I used the exercises and it worked. I've never had a problem with carpal tunnel again, and I type on the computer extensively on a daily basis.

Nervous System

My parasympathetic nervous system had been shut down for a long time, perhaps my whole life. It did not switch on and off properly. The sympathetic nervous system is the fight-or-flight mode which the body uses for handling stress. The parasympathetic nervous system is the relaxation mode which the body uses for rest and healing. Emotional trauma early in life can cause the parasympathetic system to turn off, and stay off, in an attempt to keep the body vigilant in defense against attack.

It was only in August of 2015 that a nutritionist, Joseph Strickland, was able to test my nervous system using a computer program called Nerve Express, which quantitatively measures the autonomic nervous system based on heart rate variability. This program measures the parasympathetic nervous system while you are lying down and then the sympathetic nervous system while you are standing, and shows what happens when you transition between the two. It then plots out a chart of how the nervous system is functioning compared to how it should be functioning. He determined that the reason my nervous system was not switching on and off was because my body was not producing enzymes properly. One supplement began to get things on the right track. At first, my nervous system registered the same stress lying or standing. After several months of supplementation, my nervous system registers no stress lying down, and then normal stress when standing. There is still room for improvement, but this is a big shift in the right direction.

RIFE MACHINE

I acquired a Rife machine from a Canadian company in 2004. You cannot buy them in the US. Royal Rife developed the machine in the 1920s. The machines available now are the best approximation of Royal Rife's specifications. The machine I got had a plasma tube and a minicomputer, which allows you to program series of frequencies into the machine. There is a CAFL (Consolidated Annotated Frequency List) booklet which lists the effective rife frequencies for all sorts of maladies. Many types of parasites are listed there. You can use this list to program the machine to run through all the frequencies of the parasites that you have. As parasites can mutate out of the frequency ranges, it is possible to program the computer to run through converging ranges so that the parasites cannot escape. I spent many hours sitting in front of the Rife machine while the plasma tube sent out the programmed frequencies. It does kill parasites, but it was not enough to eliminate them completely in my case. The Rife machine can be used on any illness. You just need to look up the frequencies in the CAFL booklet for any illness you want to work on.

ULTRAVIOLET BLOOD TREATMENTS

In 2013, I did several ultraviolet blood treatments. Each treatment took about ninety minutes and cost $220. A small amount of blood (enough to fill one intravenous bag) would be removed intravenously, run through a machine with ultraviolet light which kills pathogens in the blood, and then infused back into the body. The small amount of treated blood is expected to have a positive impact on the rest of the blood. I was experimenting with this procedure. It did help, but it was helping because I had a blood parasite, though I did not know that at the time. Many people use this procedure to treat Lyme bacteria in the blood. However, I had been over Lyme for eight years when I tried this treatment, so I cannot comment on its use for Lyme.

REFLEXOLOGY

Reflexology is the application of pressure to specific points on the feet, hands, or ears. It is based on the principle that nerve endings, located in the feet, hands or ears, correspond to certain body systems and organs, and applying pressure to those specific points has a beneficial effect on those organs and systems. For example, if you apply pressure to the liver point on your foot, it can stimulate energy to the liver, which can assist healing and the release of toxins. If you are taking medication for the liver, pressure on the liver point will also increase the uptake of that medication to the liver.

There are many reflexology charts on the Internet. You can find one and work on yourself. It is typical to use the thumbs to apply the pressure. You will find that the more toxic and out of balance your organs are, due to illness, the more painful a reflexology session will be.

ELECTROMAGNETIC FIELDS (EMFs)

Kinesiology has shown that EMFs are harmful to the immune system. More studies are beginning to show that the radiation from cell phone use is harmful to the brain. I rarely use a cell phone. Dr. Cowden recommended a maximum limit of 2 to 3 mG (milligauss) for an electromagnetic field that you live and sleep in. Spending a great deal of time in fields measuring higher than that can make it hard to recover from chronic illness. You can buy an EMF detector to measure the fields around your home. A cell tower or other high voltage tower with power lines typically exceeds that limit, so it would not be wise to live near one. Even telephone lines can emit powerful EMFs. Their level of harm depends on how far you live from one.

GEOPATHIC STRESS

Geopathic stress occurs when the earth's magnetic field is disturbed, either naturally or artificially, and the background field we normally experience is changed. This often occurs due to underground water currents. Geopathic stress results in concentrations of negative earth energies, which have a detrimental effect on humans and some animals.

In 1929, Gustav Freiherr von Pohl had a theory that earth energies were connected to the fact that fifty-four people in his town of Vilsbiburg, Germany, had died of cancer. He proceeded to dowse the town for stress lines and mapped his results. When he compared his map to a map of the houses where the people had died of cancer, he found that every one of those fifty-four people had slept in beds that were directly over the stress lines he had dowsed. Thus, cancer was linked with earth energies.[20]

It is possible to have your home dowsed in order to see if your bed, or any place where you spend a lot of time, is on a geopathic stress line. As with EMFs, geopathic stress interferes with immune function, so it can be difficult to heal from chronic illness if you experience this stress for long periods of time. If you have a pet, you will notice that cats like to be in areas of geopathic stress, whereas dogs will avoid them.

HOMEOPATHY

Homeopathy is a practice of diluting a substance in a solution down to very small amounts and treating illnesses with them. Some solutions are diluted to the point where no molecules of the original substance remain. All that is left is the energy of the substance, and that is what has an effect on the body.

I have not seen homeopathy used directly on an illness. It was used to resolve my jaw cavitation. Practitioners have often used homeopathics for things like stimulating lymphatic drainage. I have taken them as treatment for parasites as well. As they are energetic medicines, a practitioner could easily program other helpful frequencies into them. A practitioner using a bioresonance machine will have determined which frequencies will be helpful for your body, and these can be programmed into your bottle with the homeopathic medicine to give a variety of helpful energetic frequencies.

When it was determined that my blood was deficient in phosphorous, which allowed a blood parasite to thrive, the practitioner determined that the best way to restore the phosphorous levels to the blood was for me to take a homeopathic phosphorous liquid rather than the actual substance. The treatment worked. The blood levels of phosphorous were restored, and the blood parasite was eliminated.

EARTHING

Earthing is the practice of literally getting in touch with the earth. You can go outside and stand on the ground with your bare feet. There is something about the exchange of energy and electrons with the earth that has a beneficial effect on your body. You can buy products that you can use indoors. You can use a wristband that touches your body, and a cord that plugs into the third grounding hole at the bottom of US electrical outlets. This way you can stay connected to the earth while working or sleeping.

AIR QUALITY

Indoor air quality can be an issue. If you have a chronic illness it is best to avoid getting new carpet or new furniture. Each will release volatile organic compounds (VOC's) such as formaldehyde into your home. Formaldehyde has a negative impact on your immune system. House cleaning products typically use toxic chemicals as well.

Air purifiers are one way to deal with this problem.

Essential Oils

I used some of these only for a short time. A practitioner was finding that I tested positive for them for a while, but not for any specific purpose. I did try them for parasites with little effect. Others claim that oils are very effective for many issues. There is room to experiment here. There are practitioners knowledgeable in the use of essential oils who can assist.

Summary

I can only describe my experience with different modalities. I cannot say which ones will work the best. I wasn't often able to tell how well modalities worked for me. I couldn't really notice when a modality resolved one or two issues because so many others remained which were making me feel bad. And different things work for different people. I didn't find too many magic bullets in this illness. You have to find what works for you . . . and keep searching.

Dr. Mercola has an excellent alternative health website and a free daily newsletter that are a good way to keep up with alternative medicine (see "Resources" in chapter 5).

[5]

Summary of Physical Healing

- Many significant chronic health issues are caused by treating Lyme disease with medications that harm the gut flora (beneficial bacteria) in the intestines. By treating Lyme disease with medications that do not harm the gut flora, many of these chronic health issues can be avoided.

- If you treat Lyme disease with antibiotics, be sure to take probiotics and fermented foods in order to support your gut flora during treatment.

- I needed many testing methods to determine the many different issues I had. To do this, I had to try many practitioners from alternative and conventional medicine.

- I needed many treatment modalities to treat all the issues I had, one by one. The many practitioners I saw accomplished this. Some practitioners had good testing methods but not good treatment modalities, and vice versa. I also did a large amount of research, read many books, and experimented on my own. I had to keep coming at health issues from every angle possible.

- I needed a way to measure my progress on my health issues, because I could not measure progress based solely on how I felt. The testing modalities were used for this. This is important, because going too many years without feeling better is extremely discouraging, and that has its own toxic effect on your health.

- Alternative medicine had all the tools I needed for chronic illness, but it is not covered by insurance. Conventional medicine had only some of the tools I needed for chronic illness, but it is covered by insurance.

- Your body can heal almost anything. It has more capacity for recovery than you think. Don't give up, no matter how grim it looks. Just keep moving. You have to stay in the game.

RESOURCES

BOOKS

- *Renew Your Life* - Brenda Watson (simple explanations of how the body functions in illness)
- *The Amazing Liver and Gallbladder Flush* - Andreas Moritz (good source for doing liver flushes)
- *Timeless Secrets of Health* - Andreas Moritz (book explains a great deal about alternative health procedures)
- *Gut And Psychology Syndrome* - Natasha Campbell-McBride, MD (book talks about gut issues related to gut flora)
- *The Yeast Connection* - William Crook (talks about gut issues and Candida)
- *Root Canal Cover Up* - George Meinig (explains in detail how root canals harm your health)
- *Sweet Deception* - Joseph Mercola, DO (book tells the whole story about artificial sweeteners and the lack of oversight at the FDA)
- *Overcoming Repetitive Motion Injuries the Rossiter Way* - Rossiter, MacDonald (book offers carpal tunnel treatment through exercise only)
- *Lab 257* - Michael Christopher Carroll (story of germ warfare lab near Old Lyme, CT, where Lyme disease started)
- *The Alternative Medicine Definitive Guide to Cancer* - John Diamond, MD, Lee Cowden, MD, with Burton Goldberg (this book explains much of Dr Cowden's process of healing chronic illness)

WEBSITES

- Lyme site: **www.lymediseaseresource.com** (See Dr Cowden in "Killing Protocols" tab)
- Mercola website and newsletter: **www.mercola.com** (extensive free info on alternative medicine)
- Hulda Clark article on Ascaris parasite treatment: **www.drclark.net/the-essentials/beginners/parasites/ascaris-a-tapeworms**
- Liver flushes and gallstone site: **ww.sensiblehealth.com**
- Naturopath site showing alternative medicine modalities along with dental charts: **www.naturalworldhealing.com**
- Article on gut flora: **www.nytimes.com/2013/05/19/magazine/say-hello-to-the-100-trillion-bacteria-that-make-up-your-microbiome.html**
- Fecal transplant site: **www.thepowerofpoop.com**
- Weston Price Foundation: **www.westonaprice.org** (information on Dr. Prices' research on nutrition as it relates to dental issues)
- Root canal video (2.5 minutes) by Dr Nunnally: **www.youtube.com/watch?v=BoWWXzJuuRY**
- Information about Royal Rife and the Rife machine: **www.rife.org**
- Geopathic stress dowser in Austin: **www.geoharmony.net**

PRACTITIONERS

- **W. Lee Cowden, MD** - Chairman of the Scientific Advisory Board and Professor of the Academy of Comprehensive Integrative Medicine (www.acimconnect.com)
- **Ted L. Edwards, Jr, MD** - Physician who uses alternative and conventional medicine in Austin, TX (www.centerforhealthandhealing.org)
- **Rey Ximenes, MD** - Physician who uses alternative and conventional medicine in Austin, TX (www.tpsmc.com)
- **Harry Ramnarine, MBBS** - Doctor who uses energy medicine in Trinidad and Tobago (www.facebook.com/Ishtara-Centre-135140583227038)
- **Ralph Wilson, ND, MS** - Naturopath in Washington, D.C. (www.naturalworldhealing.com)
- **Caren Coe, ACN** - Naturopath and nutritionist in Austin, TX - uses bioresonance screening machine helpful with Lyme disease (www.carencoe.com)
- **Joseph E. Strickland, ACN** - Nutritionist in Austin, TX (www.nutritionaustin.com)
- **John Bandy, DC** - Chiropractor at Austin Holistic Health in Austin, TX (www.austinholistichealth.com)
- **James Chappell, BS** - Chiropractor in Scottsdale, AZ (www.drjameschappell.com)
- **Stuart M. Nunnally, DDS, MS** - Biological dentist in Marble Falls, TX (www.healthysmilesforlife.com)

PART II

EMOTIONAL HEALING

[6]

My Story - 2011 to 2014

I got on the spiritual path at the beginning of 2008 while my marriage was ending. The best explanation of "spiritual path" that I've heard is "a search for the truth" . . . whatever truth is. This path is not a religious one, though it does not exclude religion. It is certainly not necessary to be on a spiritual path in order to do emotional healing. It's just that this path is where I came in contact with healing modalities, and eventually came to emotional healing. I became accustomed to being around people who had intuitive abilities, so for a few years I had been using various healing modalities with intuitives. An intuitive friend of mine who works with emotional healing modalities had been suggesting for a couple of years that I begin emotional healing.

ILLNESS RECOVERY STALLS

I kept hearing from various sources how emotional issues are the root cause of all physical illness, but for whatever reason, I hadn't been drawn to it. After working on physical healing for ten years, emotional healing just seemed to be another huge project to get started on, and I didn't want to deal with it. However, by 2011, my physical healing had hit a wall. I reasoned that if emotional issues were the root cause of all illness, and I had a lot of emotional issues, then clearly physical healing treatments would only get me so far. So I then accepted that I had to get started with emotional healing in order to move forward on healing my illness.

EMOTIONAL HEALING BEGINS

I started work with my friend. She was using a healing modality called Radical Forgiveness. I found the work rewarding; however, the issues I needed help with were expanding faster than she could accommodate with that method. I came across another emotional healer using shamanic methods of energy shifting. This work seemed to accomplish more at a faster pace, and it was helping me, so I switched to that. This healer was getting close to my core issues, but could not really hit the nail on the head. So in April of 2012, I found an intuitive healer in Austin named Bart Sharp.

THREE YEAR STINT IN EMOTIONAL HEALING

Bart Sharp's work really started to get at my core issues, so I knew this was the way forward for me. I continued this work weekly for about three years. The wealth of issues we explored over that time was profound. It was an education for me in many ways. He recommended I look into the work of Alice Miller, a Swiss psychologist. I read three of her books, and her work resonated with me in a huge way. During that time I also worked with other emotional healing modalities and practitioners in between the weekly sessions with Bart. In my third year with Bart, I discovered a CD program called "The Release Technique." I found that I could work on myself with this program, because it didn't require any intuitive ability. I learned that you can process emotional energy out of your body simply by feeling your feelings in your body as they occur. This work that I was doing on my own increased the pace of the work I was doing with Bart quite a bit. Things started moving faster.

WEEKLY SESSIONS

During weekly sessions, I would go in and discuss whatever emotional issues were coming up for me that week. Bart would view my energy field psychically, and he would trace any energy disturbances back to the original issue in my life that caused the problem. He would find out the circumstances of my life at the time the issue originated and discuss it with me. We would also discuss how the issue developed throughout my life. Then he would work to shift the energy using the healing modality that he specializes in, which was Access Consciousness.

Emotional Healing versus Psychotherapy

Past Psychotherapy Work

I did some conventional psychotherapy work earlier in my life with a psychologist in response to depression. It didn't help.

After my experiment with psychotherapy failed in my twenties, I went on to do a lot of self-help work over the years. I can recall the work of Tony Robbins, among many others. Some of that work was pretty good, but nothing ever put a dent in all the emotional issues I had, let alone explain any of it.

Why Psychotherapy Wouldn't Work for Me

In reading some of psychologist Alice Miller's books, she talks about the need to get back into repressed memories to experience the emotion of those memories. This means that you cannot just remember it factually, you have to feel the emotion of it so you can grieve.[1]

There are many theories on how to deal with past painful incidents, but I am finding more and more that feeling past pain is necessary for healing. Many try to avoid feeling this pain, but we never really avoid it. The body remembers every bit of it, whether we block it from our minds or not. Avoiding our feelings is what causes all the problems in the first place. The emotional energy gets stuck in our bodies and creates problems, repeating patterns, and eventually illness. I would be all for going into memories to flush out issues, but in my case, many of the issues I experienced were at such an early age that I didn't remember any of them, so relying on my memory was not an option.

EMOTIONAL HEALING

With my situation, working with a psychic was the only way for me, not only to learn what had happened to me at a very early age, but also to get to the energy of the issues so it could be shifted.

It wasn't until my healing sessions with Bart Sharp, and reading the books of Alice Miller, that the whole picture started to become clear and my healing process really began. The healing of my physical illness also moved forward.

What I've learned over time is that emotional healing is more important to my life than physical healing, mostly because emotional issues cause illness. Long after my physical healing is complete, I will still be working on my emotional issues. The tools I discuss here are a lifelong practice that serve me well. It is now just part of my life. Emotional healing was not an added burden at all. It is the vehicle I use to continually improve my life.

[7]

How We Form
Emotional Issues

Alice Miller says that, in her experience, the cause of emotional problems is found in the infant's early mode of adapting to circumstances. When the infant's needs for respect, understanding, caring, and mirroring are not met, those needs have to be repressed, which leads to serious consequences later in life.[1]

Everybody develops emotional issues. How does this happen, and why do some have worse issues than others? The most general reason we develop emotional issues is because we were not loved the way we wanted to be as children. Even if parents are loving, the issue is created from the child's perspective of not being loved in the way the child wants. If we experience trauma as a child because we don't feel loved, we may have unpleasant feelings of rejection, hurt, abandonment, and sadness. If it keeps happening, anger, frustration, and fear get added to the list, and then the child starts forming beliefs about herself as to why this is happening such as, *Maybe I don't deserve love*, or *Maybe there is something wrong with me*. We are forming judgments.

Repeating Patterns

The trauma and our reactions to it cause a repeating pattern in our lives—situations keep occurring that cause the same reactions in us. It is almost as if our souls are giving us continuing opportunities to make the situation work out right. If we react negatively to the trauma, then we begin to establish a pattern of how we react each time the situation occurs, and we judge it. We didn't like it the first time, and then it happens again. We continue to feel the same emotions each time, and develop a real aversion for the recurring situation.

Humorous Example of a Repeating Pattern

In regard to patterns, there was a funny scene from the show *New Girl*, starring Zooey Deschanel, in 2012. Someone asked why she was so trusting of people as an adult, and the show then flashed back to a formative incident when she was a young girl. The girl is walking on the sidewalk when a seemingly creepy guy drives up in a van with no windows in the back and asks her if she would like some candy, in a malevolent tone. She innocently and excitedly replied that she would. The guy said that his grandmother made too much. And just when you're envisioning the worst possible outcome, the side door of the van opens revealing the guy's grandmother holding a nice big bag of candy that she hands to the little girl before waving goodbye.² So the girl grows up trusting people. It's a bit of an oversimplification, but not far off from how patterns and beliefs are created . . . and funny, if you have a twisted sense of humor.

Learning to Suppress Emotions

So what happens when you feel emotions that cause discomfort? Children just feel them and express them—by a tantrum or crying. Shortly afterward, they are back to normal as if nothing happened. Emotional energy overcomes them, runs through them, and leaves. Then the episode is over. But over time, you get more socialized and corrected by your parents and teachers. Expressing strong emotion is no longer acceptable, and you learn how to tone down your emotional expression. Plus, you are getting sensitized to the same painful emotions which keep happening because you judge them. So you start to suppress the emotions that cause discomfort, and you learn how to avoid them through activities that distract you. If you continue to have outbursts, or cry, your friends or classmates make fun of you. So basically, you eventually learn how to stuff your emotions in order to get along with others.

The Stuck Energy of Suppressed Emotions

Emotions come up and we cannot stop them. That's great so long as they feel good, but we consider painful emotions to be a nuisance. If you just felt them and handled them the same way you did as a child, you would let the emotional energy run through you and out of you, and you would be done with it. But now you have learned how to stuff emotions by suppressing or avoiding them. What happens then? The emotional energy that is not allowed to run through you gets stuck in your body. In your attempt to avoid a painful emotion, you get stuck with it. Well, that's not so good, but it's only one episode. But what happens when you start doing this over and over again every time painful emotions come up?

BUILDING A RESERVOIR

When you get in the habit of habitually stuffing your emotions, you begin to accumulate the stuck emotional energy of the feelings you are not allowing to run through you. This creates a reservoir of all that stuck energy of emotions that you've stuffed your whole life. It is a store of energy that you hold in your body, and it inhibits your life in many ways, especially in physical health.

This reservoir of stuck energy then becomes a source point to be triggered by future situations. What happens when repeated similar episodes occur? Emotions come up that feel painful, you remember that this has happened before, and you didn't like it. You think that this shouldn't keep happening, so you suppress the feelings or find an activity that helps you avoid feeling them. But now you have been building up that reservoir of stuck energy from all the times this has happened before. When the current situation triggers this reservoir of stuck energy, it can magnify the emotional energy of the current situation many times. Your emotions can get completely out of proportion to the current circumstance, because you have now tapped into energy that was already built up around this issue. And unless you intervene with this pattern, it will tend to get worse as life goes on, as you keep building that reservoir of stuck energy. These are your emotional issues. People will watch you completely melt down over a situation that seems very minor to them. Road rage comes to mind, as an example, where people risk their lives using their vehicles, going 70 mph, to express their rage at each other because of the simple act of one cutting in front of the other. Something's going on there that has nothing to do with someone cutting in front of someone else.

EMOTIONS, THOUGHTS & BELIEFS

This discussion of how emotional issues develop was limited to emotions for clarity, but emotions affect thoughts. So during this process, when painful emotions arise, they affect your thought process as well. If you feel bad, your thoughts become darker and more repetitive which, in turn, causes even more negative emotions, and a vicious cycle can develop. Repetitive negative thinking can lead to the formation of beliefs. Thoughts are basically meaningless. They constantly move across your mind, but your body feels and reacts to them. A thought acquires meaning when you feel an emotion due to it, and when this occurs over and over again, you then begin to form a belief such as, *This always happens; I always feel this way when that happens; I'm the type of person who . . .*, etc. Your body responds to your beliefs as if they are true, whether they have any actual validity or not.

PROCESS OF FORMING AN ISSUE

So a trauma happens early in your life as per your perception. You react to it and judge it because it is painful, which causes a repeating pattern. This pattern brings a similar episode back into your life over and over again. You've judged this type of episode as "bad," and every time it happens you now resist it. Your thoughts get stirred up, and you form some beliefs about why this is happening, and now you find ways to avoid the feelings that come up in this type of episode. Your avoidance or suppression of feeling your painful emotions each time causes emotional energy to get stuck in you. The stuck emotional energy then accumulates in your body throughout your life, which magnifies your response to similar situations each time. You now have an "issue" related to your early trauma. Intervening in this process is what emotional healing is about.

> It should be noted that if avoiding your emotions causes these problems, then feeling your emotions can be a big part of the solution.

THE EFFECT OF EARLY TRAUMA

Trauma at any time in your life can create these patterns, but the ones that happen very early in your life are the most powerful, especially if you cannot remember them. The earlier these traumas happen, the bigger their effect on your life, because your emotional development is still in its formative stages. The later in life that you begin to work on these issues, the longer the patterns have been building and ingraining themselves into your consciousness, and the larger the reservoir of stuck energy you have built up in your body, which is inhibiting your life in many ways.

EXAMPLE OF HOW AN ISSUE IS FORMED

Take, for example, an infant who is not getting the love he wants. As an infant, you may be afraid to express anger at your caregivers, because you don't want to risk the relationship—after all, it is at least providing some love. In this earliest of relationships, you can't say, "This is unacceptable. I will have to end the relationship if my needs are not met." That's not an option, so you learn how *not* to speak up at a young age because you cannot risk that most critical relationship. You can't afford to say no. You can't afford to have healthy boundaries. So as an infant, if you don't speak up and you're still not getting the love you want, what do you do? First, you try to figure out why you're not getting the love you want, and you form some beliefs about yourself like, *Maybe there is something wrong with me*, or *Maybe I'm not lovable.* These beliefs, formed so early, exist below the conscious level, and may influence you your entire life without your realizing it. What do you do next? You feel a lot of frustration and anger in private. Your thoughts run around in circles: *This is the person who was supposed to give me love. Nobody else is going to do it.* But you can't express any of this or you'll risk the relationship, so it starts to feel hopeless and the frustration builds. And then you get creative and devise ways in which to please your caregiver in order to get more of the love you need. This creates a new pattern of trying to please others, and it can form the belief that you need to earn love from others because it is not freely given. You then learn to accept relationships where you give more love than you receive in return. You now have self-worth issues. This example can all come from an infant feeling trauma simply because he has been left alone too often and not held enough. This is one example, but there are myriad combinations of traumas that cause different patterns. Later in life, these patterns surface in your relationships over and over again.

CHILDHOOD TRAUMA IS NOT ALWAYS ABUSE

It is important to note that childhood trauma, as used here, does not always mean physical abuse or some terrible behavior on the part of caregivers. Trauma is a deeply disturbing experience as subjectively perceived by the child. A child can experience abandonment issues after a parent dies. All the child knows is that someone left her.

THE STORY OF MOSES

In her book *The Body Never Lies*, Alice Miller uses the biblical story of Moses to demonstrate how the most altruistic of parental acts can cause trauma. To paraphrase that account, according to the biblical story, Moses' life was in danger as an infant, so his mother had to give him up in order to save his life. She put baby Moses into a basket and put the basket into the river in the hopes that someone would rescue the child. As an adult, Moses could say how grateful he was to his mother for saving his life, because adult Moses understood that in a rational way. However, baby Moses experienced emotional trauma. All the baby knew was that his mother had abandoned him. He must have thought, *Why did she cast me out? Did I do something wrong? Am I going to drown? Will a cobra get me? A crocodile? Will anyone ever find me? Will my mother come back for me?* He was picked up by strangers and started a new life among them, never knowing why he was abandoned by the person who was supposed to love him most. That is a traumatic experience, and the baby felt every bit of it, regardless of what the rational reasons were behind it.[3]

This demonstrates how an infant can suffer trauma in a seemingly innocent situation when a caregiver is doing the most altruistic act possible for the child. Emotional trauma has nothing to do with the rational understanding of a situation. It is simply about the emotional experience of the child. Alice Miller went on to speculate that Moses must have had some big issues, and repeating patterns, in his life relating to his early trauma.

ENERGY SPLIT IN TRAUMA

The energetic mechanism of trauma is that a portion of a person's energy splits off because it cannot handle the trauma, but it stays connected to the person. This is a way of saving and protecting that traumatized portion of energy. The only method of communication that the traumatized, split-off energy then has with the person is to force repeating behaviors. So an addiction may be the only indication of some early form of trauma. Physically, the body stores the memory of every event in its cells. It's nice to think that a baby doesn't remember any of an early traumatic experience, and so it doesn't affect him later on. However, the baby's body experienced the trauma and a portion of his energy split off, and that split-off energy is still there throughout his life, continuing to force repeating behaviors until such time as that energy is healed.

SOUL FRAGMENTATION IN NATIVE TRADITIONS

This concept of energy splitting off is similar to the concept of soul fragmentation in Native American and Shamanic traditions. They use the process of soul retrieval to call back and integrate the portion of the person's soul that fragmented during trauma. In those traditions, soul fragmentation is considered to be a cause of illness.

[8]

The Effect of Emotional Issues on Health

SCIENTIFIC STUDY

In the 1990s, a study was done called "The Relationship of Adverse Childhood Experiences to Adult Health: Turning Gold into Lead." This study was done in cooperation with 17,421 adults at Kaiser Permanente's Department of Preventive Medicine in San Diego, California, to study how childhood experiences affect adult health decades later. The average age of the participants in the study was fifty-seven years old, so they were looking at health effects fifty years later. What they found was that adverse childhood experiences, or some form of trauma, are vastly more common than thought, and that the incidence of severe illnesses were many times higher in the group of people who had suffered adverse childhood experiences than those who did not suffer those adverse experiences.[1]

So there is documented scientific evidence of the effect of childhood trauma on health. What are some ways that emotions affect health?

Early Trauma & the Nervous System

Early trauma can impact the nervous system, which can have an adverse effect on physical health. The autonomic nervous system is a part of the nervous system that controls bodily functions that are not consciously directed, such as heart rate, digestion, and breathing. This influences the function of the internal organs. The autonomic nervous system consists of two branches—the sympathetic and the parasympathetic. The sympathetic nervous system activates to respond to stressful situations and mobilize energy. It puts the body in fight-or-flight mode. The parasympathetic nervous system activates to calm the body and rest. It puts the body in relaxation and healing mode. In a healthy body, both systems activate and shut off depending on the circumstances. However, early trauma can cause the parasympathetic nervous system to turn off and stay off. The body then remains in fight-or-flight mode to keep the child hypervigilant due to fear of trauma. Over time, this constant stress takes a toll on the immune system, which uses the healing mode of the parasympathetic nervous system to maintain and repair body health.

The Effect of Emotions on Organs

Emotions can have adverse effects on the abdominal organs. According to traditional Chinese medicine, emotions have a correlation with the organs. The emotions and organs are related through the acupuncture meridian system which runs through the body, and connects to the teeth (see Dental Chart in Figures 1a and 1b in "Dental Issues" in chapter 4). So issues related to emotions, organs, and the teeth are all related energetically. The following chart shows typical correlations between emotions and the organs, though some variations are noted between sources. Also, some issues have varied effects. Depression, for example, can be considered as sadness, or as anger directed inwards. It will affect a different organ system depending on which emotion it is based on.

ORGANS	EMOTIONS
Heart	Joy
Liver	Anger
Lungs	Sadness
Spleen	Worry
Gallbladder	Shock
Kidney	Fear[2]

These emotions can have a negative impact on the corresponding organs when they are out of balance. For example, when we habitually feel anger and frustration, it takes a toll on the liver. Long-term grief and sadness will take a toll on the lungs.

ALICE MILLER'S WORK

If these emotional issues are left unresolved, they will have a negative impact on your life and can eventually lead to chronic illness. In the book *The Drama of the Gifted Child*, psychologist Alice Miller demonstrates the ways in which upbringing can cause childhood trauma which creates emotional issues.[3] In her book *The Body Never Lies*, Miller demonstrates, through case studies of the illnesses of several famous authors, how unresolved emotional issues lead to chronic illness.[4] These two books provide a good basis for understanding how emotional issues are formed and how they affect health. The books are an easy read, written in language the average person can understand, and they are not long. Together they form a practical basis for the study of emotional issues in regard to health.

THE BODY REMEMBERS EVERYTHING

In *The Body Never Lies*, Alice Miller states that the mind can be fooled by words but the body cannot. The body holds the truth of our experience over a lifetime. Through physical symptoms, the body forces us to rationally engage with our truth so that we can communicate with the child within us who was once rejected, abused, and humiliated.[5]

In other words, the body remembers every emotional wound regardless of whether your mind remembers. Your mind might be telling you everything is just fine, but your painful emotions will indicate that something more is going on. When you listen to the emotions instead of the mind, you can learn the true story, and only then can you begin to heal.

SUMMARY

Childhood trauma can turn off the part of your nervous system that allows you to rest and heal your body, which means that you stay in fight-or-flight mode for long periods of time, which is a stressful state. At the same time, the trauma causes repeating behavioral patterns throughout your life. Your reactions to these patterns trigger painful emotions which you suppress or avoid, causing the emotional energy to get stuck in your body, which has an effect on your abdominal organs and your body in general. This built-up energy inhibits all areas of your life, especially your health. This makes you a candidate for stress and chronic illness later in life. Most of this comes from events we barely remember very early in life, but our body remembers every bit of it. Our emotional issues provide the clues to pain that we suffered long ago.

[9]

Emotional Self-Study

You have been forming emotional issues all your life, and now you know that they affect your health. So what do you do?

Emotional issues are the elephant in the room that nobody wants to acknowledge in regard to healing physical illness. Emotions are the biggest causative factor in illness, yet even when people are stuck in illness, they won't look at their emotional issues when this could lead the way to healing.

WHY PEOPLE DON'T DO EMOTIONAL WORK

Most people give short shrift to emotional healing. It's a vague subject to begin with, they don't think they need it, nobody really knows how to do it, and the first thing you think of is therapy, which takes a long time and costs a lot of money. Plus, you know people who've been in therapy for years who are still as screwed up as they were before, only now they analyze everything. There is also the stigma. So how do you decide whether or not you need emotional healing? It was not easy for me to recognize, and I was the poster child for it. My romantic relationships were difficult and always ended painfully. I was depressed most of my adult life. Those are pretty obvious clues, but I had tried therapy many years before and it was no help at all. Medication for emotional issues is just covering up the problem, and it doesn't even do that well . . . or at all. So even if you realize you could use help, the typical options available are not good and they cost a lot of money. So you just go on living, like everybody else.

I Resisted Emotional Healing Also

At age forty, I got a serious chronic illness (or finally realized that I had already had a serious chronic illness for twenty-five years). It was when I had been dealing with that illness for many years that an intuitive friend suggested emotional healing to me, but it didn't seem to make much sense. Many people think that way. They'll say, "Emotional healing? Really? For me? Who wants to get into all that? What a can of worms that is. I don't want to dredge all that shit up and feel it again. That's dangerous, isn't it?" I like the last one about not wanting to feel it again, as if you aren't already doing that with all the repeating patterns in your life which replay these issues over and over. So if I couldn't see the need for emotional healing, with all that I had going on, then I guess people who don't have that many issues see even less reason for it. If you feel reasonably well, and your relationships are alright, then you might not even consider it. Or if your relationships aren't too good, you can at least blame all that on your partners. Plus, it's not like there is a lot of information available on ways to do emotional healing that are practical and cost-effective. Even on the spiritual path, not many people do this work, yet it is probably the most important work that any person could ever do.

So when my physical healing stalled in 2011, I tried the emotional work.

EMOTIONS—THE GREAT EQUALIZER

People have varying levels of ability in all areas of life, but not with emotions. Emotions are the great equalizer. You are not born with great emotional gifts. You may be an intellectual genius, gifted athletically or musically, a born charismatic leader, or spiritually advanced with extraordinary intuitive gifts, but everyone starts at the same level emotionally. Everyone feels the same emotions and struggles with anger, fear, sadness, and shame because of loss, betrayal, abandonment, heartache, etc. It's an equal playing field when it comes to emotions.

INDICATIONS OF EMOTIONAL ISSUES

What are the indications that you might need emotional work? How do your issues stack up? In many ways, your external world is a reflection of your internal world. So if you want to know what's going on inside, take a look outside—at your relationships, your interactions, your health, your job, and so forth.

Some indications of emotional issues are:

- Difficult relationships
- Repeating behaviors and addictions
- Difficulty saying no to others
- Wanting approval, the need to please others, overachievement
- Being a perfectionist, controlling
- Not feeling safe
- Depression and grandiosity
- Contempt for others
- Infidelity, betrayal and trust issues
- Feeling like a victim
- Feeling unworthy
- Sexual abuse
- Chronic health issues

All of these issues are interrelated, and they typically show up in repeating patterns. Some sort of trauma happened to you early in life, and you reacted to it in some way and focused on it, which then formed a pattern. You will find this type of pattern will repeat itself throughout your life. Have you noticed any of these patterns in your life? Learning about your patterns in relationships will tell you a lot. Have you had the same relationship over and over again, but with different people? Do you always attract the same type of romantic partners or friends? Have you been abused, abandoned, or betrayed several times? It's not a freak coincidence. You're going to have to get involved with your own healing, so self-study is a place to start.

DIFFICULT RELATIONSHIPS

Energetically, humans are like radio transmitters and receivers. Your energy field has a certain vibration, based in large part on your emotional makeup, and you transmit its frequency. You will only be attracted to people with a similar frequency—people who typically have similar emotional issues to yours. In fact, the only people that you are physically attracted to romantically are the ones in your vibrational range. Like a radio, your receiver only tunes in to people transmitting the same frequency that your receiver is on. You are not attracted to people out of your frequency range, no matter how physically attractive they may be. Have you ever seen a really attractive person that you have no interest in at all, or had a powerful attraction to someone who is not so attractive? Your transmitter works the same way, so if you have always attracted the "wrong" type of person romantically, it can be frustrating, but it is not your fault. You may even judge yourself harshly because of this, with thoughts like *I always choose people like that.* But you really do not control it. You are only attracted to this type of person because of your emotional issues, which were created early in life and based on your experience with caregivers. If you have self-worth issues, all kinds of negative beliefs about relationships, and defense mechanisms to protect yourself, you will attract someone like this also. What are the chances of that working out well? If you knew this, you could go easy on yourself and not judge yourself so much. So actually, these people you attract are not the "wrong" ones at all. They are exactly the right type of people for you to learn your lessons with. These patterns exist so that you can learn soul lessons. If you find yourself in a relationship with someone who seems really screwed up, then blaming that person won't help. The place to look for answers is within yourself—you attracted this person into your life. The way out is to learn the lessons, work on your issues, and not react so harshly every time it happens. These experiences are just here to teach you, painful as they may be, so you can grow. The pattern will keep happening, but if you work on your emotional issues, the effect is diminished and the pattern can eventually shift.

Repeating Behaviors and Addictions

Repeating behaviors are caused by early childhood trauma, as discussed previously, where a portion of the person's energy has split off and remains in distress. The only way for this distressed energy to communicate with the person is to force a repeating behavior or addiction. The addiction serves as the only indicator of early trauma that needs to be healed. Given that this indicator is not very clear, some investigation needs to be done to figure out the nature of the early trauma that caused the pattern. Addictions can sometimes be stopped by willpower, but like physical illness, sometimes the underlying emotional causes are so deep that no amount of willpower or effort will resolve it. It is important to understand the cause so that you can go easy on yourself through this process. If willpower is not working for you, it is important not to blame yourself or feel shame every time you fail. Shame will only strengthen the addiction. If you can understand the childhood trauma that caused it, and that it is not some weakness in yourself, you can find the compassion for yourself that you would easily give to someone else going through the same thing. Self-love is needed here.

Addictions are basically the avoidance process you use when painful feelings come up. Addictions typically feel good, so you use them to drown out the pain. You often do them without realizing it. However, this unconscious process does nothing to heal the underlying pain or the addiction. It is the underlying pain which is the key to resolving an addiction. The emotions of that underlying pain have to be processed. Even if you are able to stop an addictive behavior with willpower, you still haven't resolved the underlying pain which caused it—which is the real issue that needs resolution. We are familiar with the well-known addictions of drugs, alcohol, sex, etc., but when you look at addiction as avoidance, you realize that many things can be considered an addiction. If you include looking at your e-mails every five minutes on your cell phone, then most of society has an addiction. Why do people do this? To distract themselves from boredom, loneliness, or any other ache in their lives. What about exercising compulsively? Continual spiritual practices? Reading self-help books? Are you avoiding your life by compulsively trying to improve it?

To resolve this, you have to look at the underlying ache that causes you to take an action to avoid it. Then you have to process those feelings. You are often judging yourself for your weakness and feeling shame over your failure to stop a repeating behavior, but if you learned about what actually caused this as a child, you could begin to give yourself a break. That, in itself, could help stop the shame, and shame is what holds the pattern in place. It's just trauma causing a repeating behavior. The trauma was caused by some event that happened to you—it wasn't your fault. You may not even remember it, and now you're carrying around this behavior and beating yourself up over it because you can't stop it. The addictive behavior may not be related in any way to the initial trauma, but you get lost focusing on the behavior. The same family trauma could cause one person to be addicted to alcohol, and another to drugs. Yet, neither of these behaviors has anything to do with the underlying trauma. You may even join an organization for people who suffer from the same addiction, which may validate you as a person, but does nothing to resolve the underlying emotional issues. You can call the addiction a disease and take medication for it. It might lessen the stigma, but you're still not getting to the real issue.

DIFFICULTY SAYING NO TO OTHERS

If you have a hard time saying no to people, that is an example of not having good boundaries. That tells you a lot about your relationship with your early caregivers, because that is where you learned this. If you weren't happy with the situation, you couldn't say no because you were afraid to risk the relationship, so you learned how to always put others' needs before your own. After all, if you have low self-worth, then you feel lucky to even have others in your life. You don't want to risk that by saying no to them.

If you have poor boundaries and can't say no to people, you typically don't attract other people who are the same. That would be merciful. You could then be around others who are overly considerate of each other, and polite, because nobody has any boundaries or wants to offend another. It would be almost like the two gophers in the *Looney Tunes* cartoons who are so enthralled with being overly polite with each other that they don't realize grave danger is bearing down on them. Of course, you wouldn't learn much from that. No, if you have boundary issues, you will attract people driving a steamroller who will continually roll right over you until you are flattened into a doormat. They will constantly ask you for favors but will not help you in return. You think that if you do them some favors, then they will not ask for more, because that is how you would behave. But that only encourages them. When you go out socially, they only want to do what they want; your desires are never considered. You are just expected to tag along. You think they will be there when you need them, because you did that for them, but they won't be. They will talk for an hour about their problems, but if you then want to mention something bothering you, they will immediately excuse themselves and leave. You keep thinking they are just like you, but they aren't. They don't have the give-and-take gene. In fact, they don't really care about you at all. They just want what they want, and you were always there to give it to them. Make no mistake: they have their own issues that cause them to be like this. They are not necessarily bad people—you may do some of these things, too. But you have to take care of yourself. That's your job. The sad part is that this type of relationship may seem acceptable to you, because this is the same type of relationship you had with an early caregiver. To break the pattern, you first have to recognize it, and then you have to respect yourself enough to start saying no. You may not want to risk your relationship with these people, but you have to respect your relationship with yourself more. It can be hard to start saying no at first, but it gets easier with practice. It is only when you start saying no, and you see the reaction from these people that you realize how little they ever respected you in the first place. They tend to go away when you start saying no because they really weren't that interested in you anyway, and that's fine. I used to agonize over the explanations I would give people to justify saying no to them, but the explanations didn't help. They either won't care, or they'll get so angry they'll end the relationship. Your concern, and your carefully considered explanation, mean nothing.

No is a complete sentence. Nothing more is required. You not only have the right, but the responsibility to look after yourself. When you get imposed upon, how does it feel in your gut? If it doesn't feel right to you, say no.

WANTING APPROVAL, THE NEED TO PLEASE OTHERS, OVERACHIEVEMENT

This is also related to the difficulty of saying no and boundary issues. One of the reasons you hate to say no is because you want someone's approval. If you have the need to please others, that is a sign that you had to earn love as a child because it wasn't given freely. You can become accustomed to working hard for love in relationships, and you may not realize that you aren't getting as much in return. You learned this from your earliest caregivers. You got accustomed to relationships being like this, and sadly, you don't even notice anymore.

Many people become overachievers in life. Do you have multiple academic degrees, a roomful of trophies, and certificates hanging on the walls? If you believe you are not good enough, you'll keep trying to prove yourself through outward achievement. However, the achievements only fill the void briefly, so you have to keep achieving. It is the only way to feel good about yourself. You can never really rest and just enjoy life. If you never reach the goals you are chasing, perhaps you never get to see how empty a feeling it is to actually accomplish them. In my case, I reached a high enough level of success in many areas that made me realize there was nothing to it—there were no more illusions to chase in achievement. You never received love just because of who you were, and now you just keep on trying to find it outside of yourself by gaining recognition from the world. It's tiring, and you'll never reach your goal of proving your worth because it can't be found in achievement. If you pay attention to your behaviors, you will notice more and more all the little ways you try to please others. Do you agree to do things you don't want to do? Do you drive a little faster so the driver behind you won't get mad? Do you avoid speaking the truth because it might offend someone? Do you tip well in a restaurant so the waiter won't think you're cheap? Do you drop names, talk about your accomplishments, or show off your new car?

If you always try to please a partner in a relationship, you're being the flip side of a person who always tries to sexually conquer romantic partners. Both had to earn favor from an early caregiver, but the conqueror retains anger at the caregiver who was stingy with love. These seemingly opposite types are actually just two sides of the same coin. This is why people with betrayal issues attract betrayers— the vibration is similar. The underlying self-worth issues are the same. When you always try to please a partner because you don't feel good enough, you will typically attract partners who are unimpressed by your efforts. They don't believe you're good enough either, but you never stop trying. If you always sexually conquer others because you don't feel good enough, you will typically attract someone who is desperate for your love, but you only give it briefly . . . before your anger kicks in, causing you to reject the conquest. Then you conquer another to repeat the cycle.

Being a Perfectionist, Controlling

If your environment felt out of control to you as a child, you may spend the rest of your life in the repeating pattern of trying to control your environment. Were you always corrected when your efforts were a little in error? Were your efforts never quite good enough to get that approval you so desperately craved? So now you strive to do things perfectly. You're still trying to be good enough, to get that approval you didn't get as a child. Maybe if you do a little better this time, you'll get that approval. A roomful of trophies won't fill that void.

The adults in your life, as you grow up, love the fact that you are a perfectionist. Everybody talks about what a good little worker you are, how conscientious you are, and how you'll go far in life. You may go far in life externally, because you feel the need to prove your worth, but it's not really coming from a good place. The unfortunate thing is that we really don't control our circumstances. Sometimes things work out the way we want and it gives us the illusion that we can control some of it, but mostly life just happens. Maybe we don't control any of it. So perfectionism, in pursuit of gaining perfect outcomes, is really a hopeless cause. As far as the approval you crave, you will get some, but it will never fill the void enough to replace the love you didn't get as a child.

The story of chess champion Bobby Fischer, at the 1972 World Chess Championship, is an example of controlling behavior gone berserk, played out on a world stage. Fischer had a chaotic childhood. At the 1972 championship, he was overwhelmed by the fanfare and lost the first match on a foolish move. He didn't show up for the second match and forfeited. Fischer then set almost impossible conditions for his continued play, such as playing the match in a small room in the basement with no TV cameras, among many other bizarre conditions. Amazingly these conditions were met. He then played brilliantly and won. After that, he forgot about all the conditions. He just needed them to gain total control of the situation in order to regain his composure and play well.

NOT FEELING SAFE

If you experienced a birth trauma, the first belief you may have formed in this life is, *This world is not safe.* You won't remember it, but it may stay with you the rest of your life and color the way you view everything. Your nervous system may have been impaired right from the start. There are any number of traumas you could experience as a child that would also cause you to not feel safe. As with the issue of being controlling, your childhood could have felt chaotic and you never felt safe. This is all related to trust issues, which will again play out in relationships later in life. Do you feel safe in relationships? If you've been betrayed a number of times, probably not.

DEPRESSION AND GRANDIOSITY

Alice Miller claims that depression and grandiosity are both used to manage the pain of never having been loved for who you really are. Depression is the defense against the deep pain over the loss of the self that results from shutting down one's feelings, and grandiosity is the defense against depression.[1]

Healthy self-esteem is based on being able to feel your own authentic feelings. If you learned to shut down your feelings as a child in order to conform to the wishes of your parents, then your self-esteem did not develop properly. Perhaps your parents were embarrassed if you cried. Maybe they shamed you for complaining when others were worse off than you. Or maybe you just sensed that your need for affection stressed out your mom, so you never asked for it. Whatever the reason for shutting down your feelings, the way you then constructed your self-esteem was through external qualities such as looks, intelligence, talents, or achievements. You received admiration for your gifts and came to depend on it. This need for approval is a poor substitute for the love you didn't get as a child, but it is all you have. However, this false self-esteem work-around is dependent on your external qualities and others' admiration of them. It is a house of cards which will crumble when one of those qualities fails. When the grandiosity defense fails, it leads to severe depression. You may not realize your self-esteem was built on such a flimsy foundation, but the crash will educate you.

Alice Miller talks about people who were the pride of their parents and should have had a strong sense of self-assurance, but they didn't. So long as they were on top, the center of attention, they were fine, but when the grandiosity defense fails and they are no longer the superstar, they feel like failures and are plagued by anxiety, shame, and guilt.[2] Many performers have claimed to have been on top of the world on stage during a show, only to reach the depths of despair after they went home.

Feeling your original feelings from childhood (if you can access them), and grieving over them, is the place to start the healing. Once you learn how to feel again, authentic self-esteem and humility can emerge.

CONTEMPT FOR OTHERS

Contempt for others is another defense mechanism you develop for avoidance. Alice Miller makes the case that the function of all forms of contempt is the defense against unwanted feelings.[3] So when looking at addiction as the actions we habitually take to avoid unpleasant feelings, contempt would be a common one. In order to have contempt, you need to demonstrate your superiority over another. So a good deal of your time and effort must be devoted to comparing yourself to others and determining how you are better. Gossip would fall into this category. Making others wrong in order to show that you are right is at the heart of most arguments: "You did such and such to me, but I don't do that to you." This implies that you are wrong and I am superior, because I don't do what you do.

If you believe you are unlovable unless you are superior in some way, then you go back to building that self-esteem house of cards based on your external qualities. This ties in with having to earn your parent's love—you have to be good enough first. The easiest way to be good enough, then, is to be better than others. You can be better than others by either elevating yourself or by putting others down, although either leads to the same false place.

If you're gifted and have proven that you have superior qualities over another, what does that imply? It implies that you are worthy of love and the other is worthless. But upon further examination, if love is based on superior qualities, then without your superior qualities, you could never be loved either. If you are loved only for your gifts, then you are not really loved at all. And you can lose those gifts, so now you have to keep proving your superiority . . . partly through contempt.

If you are the grandiose gifted person, you do not have to resort to putting other people down in order to set yourself above them. Your gifts allow you to naturally elevate yourself above others. So not only do you have your natural contempt for others, but you can also consider yourself superior even to those who put others down—the gossipers. You can be contemptuous of the contemptuous, all the while playing the same game. You are pretty much superior to everyone. This is not just adding more rooms onto your self-esteem house of cards, now you're adding new floors as well. The higher you build it, the harder it will crash. With natural gifts and talents, it is almost as if God has given you as much rope as you need to hang yourself.

Being humble isn't some pretense at denying your true worth. It is the result of healing the underlying cause of what makes you want to puff yourself up in the first place—the pain of not being loved simply for who you were as a child. When you heal that, you develop true humility and self-esteem.

INFIDELITY, BETRAYAL, AND TRUST ISSUES

When we are betrayed, we typically blame the person who betrayed us. That seems reasonable on the surface. However, the emotional issue of betrayal is already within us from some childhood trauma, and we attract people of the same vibration. These are not necessarily people with the exact same emotional issues. People who have been betrayed do not typically attract others who have been betrayed, so that they can commiserate and comfort each other. That would be merciful, but we wouldn't learn much from that. If you have betrayal issues, you typically attract people who will betray you . . . again and again. There are usually strong victimization and self-worth issues involved, so you will attract someone who will victimize you, given that you feel you deserve it. After being betrayed several times, which only strengthens the self-worth and victimization issues, you may develop a disgust for romantic partners altogether. The lesson to learn here, though, is that it was not at all about the romantic partners. It was about the betrayal issues inside you which caused you to attract these types of people. However, it was only due to some trauma that happened to you as a child which created these issues. A caregiver may have betrayed you in some way. It had nothing to do with you, but you formed some beliefs about it and now you carry this pattern. You may now feel bad about yourself because of it, and resent all your lovers and even love itself. To realize that these issues are in you and that you attracted these people is actually empowering, because you can do something about it, and you can stop blaming others. You can do emotional healing work.

Life and relationships are not random. We are not victims. Some people get betrayed over and over. Others never do, because they don't have betrayal issues. Some people are betrayers. Others never do it. When you learn about these issues, you begin to realize that the betrayers also have similar issues from similar traumas in their childhoods. It helps you have compassion for them as well as yourself.

FEELING LIKE A VICTIM

Feeling like a victim is thinking you are helpless and at the mercy of all the people and circumstances in your life. This is evidenced by how much you blame others, and it adds to your contempt for others. Victimization can be a behavior learned from early caregivers who believed themselves to be victims and constantly complained. It can also come from traumas that happened too often before you could adequately process them, so you formed beliefs about powerlessness because that was your experience. It helps to understand that your external experience is a reflection of your internal state. Then you can begin to look inward and dismantle the faulty beliefs that keep you believing you are powerless, which will affect the external circumstances in your life. This is related to all the issues on this list.

FEELING UNWORTHY

Feeling unworthy is one of the most common emotional issues, and is related to most of the other issues on this list. When early trauma occurs, the child is not emotionally mature enough to handle it in a balanced way. If a three-month-old infant is left alone too often, the infant does not recognize that this is just a parent having a hard time. The infant only knows it has a strong need that is not being met, and may begin to form negative beliefs like, *There's something wrong with me, I'm unlovable,* or *This is my fault.* These beliefs, which reside well below the conscious level, may govern your feelings about yourself your whole life. If you have self-worth issues, you will attract romantic partners with self-worth issues also. If you think you are not worth much, you will attract partners who treat you as if you are not worth much. If you think you are unlovable, you will attract partners who are unavailable to love you, either due to a busy career, because they are married, or who are emotionally incapable of love. These types of issues can lead to betrayal and abandonment.

SEXUAL ABUSE

When the issues of unworthiness are quite serious, you may be ripe for attracting sexual abuse. When you don't get the love you need at an early age, you can spend the rest of your life desperately looking for it outside of yourself. If you believe you are not good enough, you learn how to please others to be accepted. This desperate need for love and the desire to gain approval from others, combined with the lack of boundaries, and maybe even some shame issues around sex, are the energetic siren call for abusers everywhere. They are vibrationally drawn to their prey.

The sad part of it is that none of this is your fault. It is just something that happened to you at an early age. Not loving you the way you wanted may have been completely unintentional on someone's part. The caregivers did what they did, but you were actually the one who formed the negative beliefs about yourself in response to what the caregivers did. But are you going to be hard on yourself for coming to some poor conclusions when you were two months old? It was your only way to cope. You did what you had to in order to survive.

CHRONIC HEALTH ISSUES

As mentioned previously, childhood trauma causes emotional issues which lead to chronic health issues. This was demonstrated in *The Body Never Lies* by Alice Miller, with her case studies of the illnesses of several famous authors, and also in the scientific study "Turning Gold into Lead" mentioned previously. Therefore, the presence of chronic health issues is an indication of underlying emotional issues.

> *In looking at all these issues, it's helpful to realize that everybody is doing the best he can from his own level of consciousness.*

OBSERVING YOUR PATTERNS & TRIGGERS

In regard to emotional self-study, you first need to observe your patterns. Then you need to be aware of the things that trigger your emotions. What you really want, though, is to get at the actual issue underlying it all. The trigger is usually not the underlying issue. It seems like it is because it appeared to cause the emotions that came up, but the emotional energy was already within you. For example, if you have a fear of public speaking, the fear might not have anything to do with public speaking. You may have been punished severely for speaking out as a child, and the thought of speaking now triggers that stuck emotional energy from the childhood event. You can be a brilliant writer and have great ideas to convey, but every time you get up to speak, a paralyzing fear overtakes you. It seems reasonable to conclude that you have a fear of public speaking, but in reality, it's the energy of the childhood event that is being triggered, not the current situation. Until you process the energy from the childhood event, you will always fear public speaking. All the practice in the world won't help. On the other hand, if you address the emotional energy from the childhood event, you might find that your fear of public speaking magically vanishes. The fear was only related to the childhood experience, not public speaking. You projected the fear onto public speaking thinking it was the cause, when it was only the trigger. So when examining your own issues, always keep looking for the issue underlying what is going on at the surface.

All the issues listed in this chapter are interrelated. Different people have different issues, and to varying degrees, but I find these issues to be fairly common among those with chronic illness. Again, whenever you experience these patterns and painful emotions occur, trying to avoid or suppress them causes the emotional energy to get stuck in your body. This builds up a reservoir of stuck energy in your body. Emotional healing attempts to dissipate this reservoir or drain the swamp, so to speak. So how do we do emotional healing?

[10]

Emotional Healing Modalities

There are many emotional healing modalities. Listed here are some I have worked with:

- **Access Consciousness** - This is a healing modality which uses clearing statements to shift energies. You typically work with an intuitive practitioner who uses this modality. He or she asks questions to bring up energies that need to be cleared, and then uses the clearing statements.
- **EFT (Emotional Freedom Technique)** - This involves tapping certain points on your face and upper body while making certain statements. It helps reprogram your energy in regard to issues. You can learn this technique online for free. It is easy to learn, and you can do this on yourself.

- **Family Constellations** - This is an approach for revealing the hidden dynamics in a family so they can be
  worked with and healed. The technique involves family
  interaction through the use of others playing the roles
  of family members. The interaction is guided by a practitioner, and the interactions are revealing.
- **Grief Counseling** - You list out all your traumas in life,
  and you forgive everybody (especially yourself) and every situation. You typically go through this process with
  a counselor.
- **Healers** - There are any number of intuitive healers who
  do emotional healing work, using any number of modalities. Most intuitives have taken standard healing
  modalities and customized them to fit their own
  unique abilities. As with any practitioner, you will have
  to try some and see how they work for you.
- **Hypnotherapy** - There are different types of hypnotherapy. The type I did was where I remained conscious and
  the therapist took me through a guided meditation
  where I had direct experiences with my subconscious
  mind that unlocked certain issues that were bothering
  me and I would gain insights.
- **Ho' oponopono** - A Hawaiian method of saying four
  statements over and over again regarding any issue.
  These are: "I love you. I'm sorry. Please forgive me.
  Thank you." These statements are addressed to the Divine within you. Ho'oponopono is based on the
  knowledge that anything that happens to you or that
  you perceive, and the entire world where you live, is

your own creation and thus, it is entirely your responsibility. You heal yourself by recognizing that whatever comes to you is your creation or the outcome of bad memories buried in your mind. By regretting whatever errors of body, speech, and mind caused those bad memories, and by requesting divine intelligence within yourself to release those memories, you can set yourself free. Dr. Hew Len healed a ward of mentally ill criminals with this method without ever talking to any of them.[1] Constant repetitive usage of this method is needed.

- **Integrated Energy Therapy** - This is a healing method which uses angels to clear emotional blockages. You typically do this modality with an intuitive who specializes in IET.

- **Pranic Healing** - This is a healing modality which works on the energy field of the body. A healer will use hand motions to pull out dirty energy from a person's body, and then infuse light back in. Pranic psychotherapy is a type of Pranic healing that works to resolve emotional imbalances. In Austin, and other cities, there are free clinics where you could sample this modality.

- **Psychotherapy** - This is standard counseling with talk therapy. If you are able to bring up the unpleasant feelings from painful episodes in your life, this work can be helpful.

- **Radical Forgiveness** - This involves a standard worksheet on which you define the issue and work through all the questions on it. They are geared toward leading you to understand how this issue has served you so that you can resolve it. You can do this on your own, though it can be more powerful if you work with an intuitive.

- **Release Technique** (also called the Sedona Method) - This is a product you can buy for $280 and use by yourself. You choose an issue to work on and ask a series of questions in a certain order to bring up feelings in your body regarding that issue. You consciously feel the feelings that come up in your body until they dissipate. This works off the emotional energy around the issue. This process works on the lower three chakras (energy centers of the body). The program is a ten CD set, though I never made it past CD #3. Once I learned the original method, I just used it over and over again on hundreds of issues. This method was invented by Lester Levenson. He was in his forties, had severe heart problems, and was told he had only a few months to live. He invented this method, used it on himself, and became enlightened within three months. He lived for another forty years.

- **The Energy Programs of Panache Desai** - He offers ten-day and twenty-one-day programs during which he sends energy which will bring up emotional issues to be processed out of your body. These programs can be very challenging, as you feel all your issues come up until the program ends. Panache also does online seminars, in which he talks about emotional issues and how to deal with them (some of this work is discussed in chapter 20).

- **The Work of Byron Katie** - This involves using a standard worksheet from which you continually ask questions which examine your thoughts and motivations to break down the lies and false beliefs which cause your suffering.
- **Theta Healing** - This is a healing method which shifts beliefs. You typically do this with an intuitive who specializes in Theta healing.

Like any physical treatment modality, you have to try some of these to see what works for you. The ones that allow you to get at the energy of the issue are best, because that is what you are trying to shift. I would caution against modalities that claim you can resolve all your issues without feeling anything. There are those that claim it is harmful to revisit painful past feelings, but my opinion is that it may be necessary. Some methods can shift your energy without a lot of pain, but be cautious. Pain is part of life and its lessons. You're not meant to bypass it completely.

MODALITIES & PRACTITIONERS

MODALITIES YOU CAN USE WITHOUT AN INTUITIVE

It is not necessary to use an intuitive in the emotional healing process. The following modalities can be done without an intuitive: EFT, psychotherapy, family constellations, grief counseling, hypnotherapy, Ho' oponopono, Pranic healing, Radical Forgiveness, the Release Technique, and The Work of Byron Katie.

Modalities You Can Use Without a Practitioner

It is not even necessary to use a practitioner. The following modalities can be done on your own, without a practitioner: EFT, Ho' oponopono, Radical Forgiveness, the Release Technique, and The Work of Byron Katie. Also, in chapters 20 and 21, two more methods of working on your emotional issues are presented which you can do on your own.

Modality Cost

As for cost, some of the above modalities are free of cost, like EFT, Ho' oponopono, Radical Forgiveness, and The Work of Byron Katie. The methods presented in chapters 20 and 21 are free of cost as well. The Release Technique program costs $280, but you own the program and can use it whenever you like. The rest of the healing modalities have varying costs. You can also learn some of the modalities mentioned above and perform them yourself.

[11]

How Does a Healing Modality Work?

A healing modality works by dissipating the reservoir of stuck energy in your body due to your emotional issues. All the feelings that you have been suppressing or avoiding all your life have caused all that emotional energy to get stuck and to build up in your body. This is the energy that has manifested your illness, so processing that energy out of your body is the goal. This will clear the energy in your field and raise your vibration. It will directly improve your health.

WHAT DOES PROCESSING ENERGY MEAN?

When we discuss processing emotional energy out of the body, it may sound like an esoteric concept, but it is actually something that you are already familiar with. If you have ever grieved and been overwhelmed with sadness, you know that when you cry a great deal, it makes you feel better. This would be an example of processing emotional energy out of your body. You intuitively know this. You just don't typically refer to it as energy.

WHAT WORKED FOR ME

There were three major things that worked to process my energy over the last few years.

HEALER SHIFTED MY ENERGY

During the three years of working with the emotional healer Bart Sharp, he worked in my energy field using psychic vision and his intuitive ability to shift the stuck energy of my emotional issues. At times he would clear energy, releasing it out of me, and sometimes he would transmute a portion of the energy into a different form and reintroduce it back into my body. This all worked to raise the vibration of my energy. I was able to notice behavioral shifts over time. This was the only work that helped me actually learn about the emotional issues I had, and what had caused them, in addition to processing the energy.

DISSIPATING MY ENERGY BY FEELING IT

In the third year that I worked with Bart, I started using a program called The Release Technique on my own. In this program I would ask certain questions, in a certain order, about an issue of my choosing, which would elicit feelings in my body. By consciously observing these feelings in my body without judgment, I could dissipate the stuck energy of the emotional issue.[1]

The body is an amazing energy dissipater. All you have to do is consciously feel your feelings. To feel consciously means to focus on the area of your body where the feelings are, and to just feel the physical sensation without judging it. I would sit with these feelings in my body until they went away. No special intuitive abilities are needed for this. Anyone can do it. All you need is the willingness to dig into your own issues. This is the most straightforward way of draining the reservoir of stuck energy in your body. You just have to keep working at it, issue after issue.

SPECIALIST SENDS ENERGY TO STIR EMOTIONS

In 2015, I worked with a spiritual teacher named Panache Desai. (His teachings on nonresistance are described in greater detail in chapter 20 of this book.) Panache is known as a vibrational transformation specialist. He does energy programs on the Internet, which help detoxify the stuck energy of your emotional issues. He sends out energy which will stir up your issues, and bring that stuck energy to the surface to be processed. This occurs daily over the course of the program. You will feel your emotional issues daily during this process which can be quite challenging.

The first twenty-one day program I did had a dramatic effect. It started for me when I signed up a week before the program began. I had a significant depression that lasted for five weeks. This included the week before the program, the entire twenty-one-day program, and then the week after the program was over. That was thirty-five days of experiencing a tsunami of all my emotional issues coming forth to process out of me, and that was after three years of doing emotional work. So these programs can be quite challenging, though usually not that dramatic. I've done six other similar programs since then. Most were mild. Some had difficult periods, but not like the first one. You can receive help during those programs by calling in during webcasts. They are good programs, but not a free ride—you will have to experience your issues.

My Experience with Various Modalities

The previous three methods were how the most effective healing modalities have worked for me. Through different means, they all got to the energy of my emotional issues and started to detoxify the stuck energy from my body. This helped clean out my energy field. Whether a practitioner was using his abilities to process my energy, or I was processing it myself just by feeling my feelings, the reservoir of the stuck energy of my emotional issues was being dissipated.

I also used the other modalities mentioned in the last chapter. Counseling didn't work for me because I couldn't remember back far enough to access the feelings of those memories. It might be useful for you if you can remember your past experiences and are able to feel the emotions of them. I thought grief counseling was pretty good. You come to some interesting conclusions as you examine your life. I took part in one family constellation as a role player. The interaction was inspired and helpful to the person whose family we were modeling. EFT didn't help me much, but I know it helps a lot of people. It requires you to work on the issues that you select. I believe Radical Forgiveness and The Work of Byron Katie to be solid programs. Like the Release Technique, they are methods developed to facilitate your delving into your own issues to figure them out. If you have to select your issues to work on, then this implies enough self-awareness on your part to know your issues. How do you come to know your issues? You can work with a practitioner to explore this, or you can do the self-study work discussed in chapter 9.

Working on Your Own Issues

Learning Lessons

Working on your own issues is critical. If you are here to learn lessons in this life, then it is not likely that someone will be able to wave a magic wand and whisk away all your issues for you without your participation. That would defeat the purpose of learning. It's helpful to be aware of what issue you are trying to resolve, why you have this issue, and what you are doing to resolve it. Not many people want to do this work, but that's the whole point of being here in this life. Life is going to keep bringing you the same "learning opportunity" until you take notice and learn the lesson. If you don't take notice, the learning opportunity will become more severe each time until you get the hint. Who knows? You might even wind up with a severe illness. Finally life has your attention. Maybe now you will get to work learning your lessons . . . or not. In any case, your active participation in learning your life lessons, with the intention to resolve them, is what moves you forward on this path. When you accept the learning process, the universe will bring you the practitioners, modalities, and insights you need. If you resist, you get no help. If you treat your illness as some nuisance that you just want to get over with, then you're not getting the lesson. You have to get deeply involved.

I may have gone into emotional healing for the purpose of assisting the physical healing of my illness, but it is clear now that my healing path involved so much more than just healing an illness. You have to consider that your path may be the same. Your illness is not a nuisance to be quickly dispatched with medication. There is a purpose to it, and it may be more involved than you realize. And emotional healing may be an integral part of it.

What I Do Currently

Currently I sit down in meditation and consciously recall memories of experiences in my life that were painful or annoying—basically anything that still triggers me. Then I just sit there and feel the unpleasant sensations that come up in my body without judging them. I focus on the part of my body where I feel these feelings. I do this until the feelings are gone. This is similar to the work I did with the Release Technique.

As I am running out of memories to process, I am now focusing on facebook. On those occasions when someone posts something that annoys me, I use that opportunity to process unpleasant emotions.

When I do these practices, I feel like I am opening a spigot and letting emotional toxins drain from my body. (A more detailed explanation of this process is given in chapter 20.)

TAKE IT ONE DAY AT A TIME

Here's a newsflash: you will never be done with learning, growing, and improving yourself. Everybody on the planet is going through his or her own learning path, whether he or she has Lyme disease or not. So don't be afraid to get started with emotional healing work. It's not a big project that you will have to finish. It's something that can become a rewarding part of your daily life in addition to healing your illness.

> *If you looked at all the food you had to eat for the rest of your life in one big pile, it would be overwhelming. But when you get used to eating a few meals every day, it's no problem at all.*

[12]

Emotional Healing of Specific Health Issues

During weekly sessions with the emotional healer, Bart Sharp, I was typically working on whatever emotions were coming up during the week of the session and tracing those back to their origins. I was working on clearing a wide swath of stuck energy from my childhood that underlies all my life's emotional issues. These have affected my relationships, my emotional state, and my health. However, there were times when I would work on a specific health issue and clear the energy in regard to that. When you work on a health issue on the physical level, you treat the physical symptoms. When you work on a health issue on the emotional level, you find the emotional issues underlying the health problem and work on resolving those. Sometimes when you clear the underlying emotional issue, the physical health problem will clear up on its own.

So how do you find the emotional issue underlying a health problem? An intuitive can help with that. There are also books written on the subject. Louise Hay wrote a book called *Heal Your Body A-Z*, which lists many physical illnesses and their underlying emotional causes.[1] Written sources can sometimes provide differing accounts, but the information is usually quite good. These sources provide a quick reference to see what emotional issues may be at work in your body.

Parasites

Parasites have been an especially big issue for me. According to most sources, the underlying emotional issue is giving your power away. Giving your power away is tied to many issues—self-worth, victimization, powerlessness, boundary issues, and trying to please others. Boundary issues mean you have trouble saying no. When someone asks you for a favor, you are inclined to do it to please the person, even if it encroaches on your well-being in some way. It's related to self-worth issues. You value yourself less than others.

I have found that if you have internal parasites, then you also have external parasites . . . the two-legged kind. These are the people who take advantage of you because you let them. They like the fact that you do more for them than they do for you. They feed off you like a parasite and do little in return. When you begin respecting yourself and stop letting them do this, they tend to go away. (See the section "Difficulty Saying No to Others" in chapter 9.) Resolving these emotional issues helps to resolve the physical parasite problem as well.

EMOTIONAL ISSUES UNDERLIE PHYSICAL ILLNESS

This type of situation demonstrates the fact that emotional issues underlie physical illness. If parasites were just a physical issue, then you would have internal parasites, treat them with physical medications, and that's it. But the fact that you also have parasitic relationships with people indicates that this involves emotional issues as well as physical ones. The whole point of my journey into emotional healing was because I hit a wall in physical healing and could not go farther. Physical medications can only do so much. If the emotional issues underlying a health problem are severe enough, then all the physical medication in the world will not resolve the problem. Such was my case with parasites.

THE BODY NOTIFIES YOU

In the section "The Body Remembers Everything" from chapter 8, we discussed Alice Miller's comment that the body brings forth symptoms to demonstrate emotional wounds that your mind may not remember. Your physical parasitic infection is giving you a clue that you had an early emotional wound. If you examine your emotional issues around parasites you can see that you also have parasitic relationships in your life with people. These issues can lead you to discover the nature of the early emotional wound.

You may not remember an early wound, but the body will give you a clue.

If you have illness of any type your body it is letting you know that something is not right in your emotional world.

URINARY TRACT INFECTION

Another example of working on a specific health issue was that I developed a urinary tract infection (UTI) in 2014. This occurred while I was doing some deep emotional work on some childhood issues. I went through many natural physical protocols to heal it during that year, but none eliminated it completely. It was close to resolving a few times, but every time I did further emotional work on the same emotional issues that triggered it, the physical UTI problem flared up again. After going through every known alternative medicine treatment for the UTI, I could have given up and taken an antibiotic to stop the infection. However, I knew that the UTI would just return after treatment if the underlying emotional problem had not been cleared up as well. Plus, the antibiotics would only destroy my gut flora. Therefore, I decided to just maintain the UTI with a cranberry supplement to keep it at bay until the emotional issue worked itself out. When that happened, the physical problem cleared up.

Patience is needed. The body and emotions heal in their own time, not yours. If you panic and force a solution, it may make matters worse. Again, if the underlying emotional issue is strong enough, no amount of medication will resolve a health problem.

[13]

Personality Disorders

We don't exist in a vacuum. When we decide to heal our-selves emotionally, we don't withdraw from the world and live in a secluded healing cocoon until the process is fin-ished. We live in a changing world where unexpected events happen and we have constant interactions with oth-ers. These interactions are where we formed our emotional issues to begin with, and they continue unabated, even when we are trying to heal them. So you are not immune from continuing to interact with toxic people just because you decide to heal yourself. This is part of the challenge. However, there are certain types of people who are ex-tremely toxic. It is wise to become aware of them and learn to recognize them. You may find that you have a knack for attracting them due to your emotional issues. People with personality disorders can fall into this category. Of course, this issue is not black and white. Many, including ourselves, have varying levels of the same issues as people with personality disorders. The level of toxicity varies.

PERSONALITY DISORDER TYPES

There are different types of personality disorders. Some common ones are borderline personality disorder, narcissistic personality disorder, and obsessive-compulsive personality disorder. Some of the traits of each overlap with others. The bulk of my personal experience has been with the narcissistic personality disorder (NPD), and I will discuss that here. This is my own personal take on this subject.

NARCISSISTIC PERSONALITY DISORDER

The importance of this issue is that people with NPD can suck the life out of you. If you are in a relationship with one, it will harm your health. You will need to get away in order to heal. Loving them more does not help. Doing emotional healing work on your relationship will not help. Counseling won't help. Fortunately, narcissists won't go to counseling, because of course, they don't believe they need to. So at least you won't waste years trying to work on a relationship in counseling, thinking you are making progress when it was never possible. If you are trying to recover from Lyme disease or chronic illness, you must get away from these people. People have told me it is possible for a narcissist to change, though I've only heard of one who did, and he runs a website with his wife. Other than that one person, I've never seen one who even wanted to change. In fact, they don't even accept that they need to change. They will not discuss the issue. Needless to say, pointing out to people that they are narcissists is not wise.

Narcissism, in the common vernacular, implies a person who is egotistical, but that is not necessarily the case. Narcissism is a much deeper issue, with traits that can be very difficult to recognize. The traits can seem random, and you would have no idea that they were related in any way. There are also varying degrees to which a person can be narcissistic. This could be considered as on a spectrum, say from 0 to 100. A "normal" person might be at around 25 on the spectrum of narcissism. People who have parents with narcissistic issues will be a bit higher, say 35, and people with the actual disorder might be around 75 or higher (these numbers are for illustration purposes only and don't represent any test sampling). Everyone else falls somewhere on the spectrum. Keep in mind that US culture in the year 2015 has become quite narcissistic.

TYPES OF NARCISSISTS

There are two types of narcissist: the cerebral and the somatic. Cerebral narcissists use their intellect to manipulate others. Somatic narcissists use their bodies to manipulate others through sex.

WHY NARCISSISTS MANIPULATE

Narcissists are the ultimate manipulators. Their whole life is a manipulation. They did not develop this intentionally. At a very young age, the lack of love they received was so debilitating for them that they had to rewire their brains to create a different model of love—self-love—so they could survive. Of course, this was not real self-love. It was some sort of mental construct of self-love that permitted them to think they were so wonderful that they didn't need the love of others. Imperfect as this mental work-around was, it allowed them to survive. But it has kept them from ever looking inward at their real issues.

They will avoid most anything that makes them feel bad or might cause them to look inward at their real issues. They feel out of control in their world, and to make themselves feel more in control, they manipulate people. They will attack you and put you on the defensive. Making you the problem distracts them from looking at themselves. Blaming others gives them a sense of control over their circumstances.

WHY WE ATTRACT NARCISSISTS

As discussed earlier, we attract people of the same energetic vibration, but not necessarily of the exact same problem. Narcissists don't typically attract narcissists, though it does happen. Typically, codependent people attract narcissists. The codependents have typically had parents who had narcissistic issues, if not the actual disorder itself. So their role models for relationships were narcissists, and they spent their lives learning how to cater to and serve the narcissists in order to keep the peace. They learned early on that when a narcissist is upset, everyone will feel the wrath. So this peacekeeping behavior is what they know. It is what they are accustomed to.

When the codependent meets the narcissist, the charms of the narcissist can be overwhelming. Powerful feelings of infatuation ensue which are irresistible. To the codependent, this is the recognition of the familiar behaviors of the parent who never gave the love that was longed for. The codependent believes, however, that this new person is the one who will finally provide that long sought-after love. However, the narcissist is completely incapable of providing love. Eckhart Tolle would describe this as the meeting of two people whose pain bodies complement each other. At first it feels like heaven. Later on, it's more like hell.[1]

TRAITS OF NARCISSISTS

The interesting thing about this personality disorder is that the traits are not easily recognizable to the untrained eye. The behavior traits are strange and seemingly unrelated, yet you know something is not right. A brief summary of some of the behavior traits are that narcissists lack empathy. They can be cruel; if you bring this to their attention it will start an argument and then they become more cruel—reasoning with them does not work. They contradict themselves, sometimes in mid-sentence. They can argue one side of an issue for hours, and then suddenly change to the other side without even realizing the massive contradiction. If you present them with facts to contradict a statement they made earlier, they will say that they never said it, even if it is written down. Narcissists are harshly critical of other people, yet extremely sensitive to criticism themselves. In fact, this is an understatement. There are no gradations in this.

Even the slightest criticism of a narcissist will mean to him that you are calling him the worst person in the world. They typically lack a sense of humor; they don't really understand jokes or cartoons. Narcissists are grandiose yet naive. They don't know how things work in the world. They believe getting ahead in life is just a matter of who you know and playing the game and, of course, being the special people they are, they are among the inside players. They believe they are exempt from the same rules that everybody else has to play by, as if they are royalty. Narcissists also have strange work habits. They tend to measure the worth of their work only by how much time they spend on it, not by what they produce.

This is just a superficial description of some of the traits of narcissists. There is a good website on narcissism by Joanna Ashmun, a layperson with extensive experience in this issue. It would be wise to read the full page on her site, "Traits Discussed."[2] (Her website is listed in "Resources" in chapter 17.) If you are attracting people like this, it's time to become aware so you can work on your own issues and stop attracting them.

How to Stop Attracting Narcissists

It is always good to start becoming aware of these emotional issues, but what I have learned is that once you spot one of these people, you can't just run away. If you have attracted this person with NPD into your life and you run away, then you will just attract another. This will continue until you resolve the issues in you that attracted them in the first place. In fact, you probably already have others like them in your circle of friends and family, you just haven't realized it yet. So on the one hand, there are some people you need to get away from, but on the other hand, you will need to be patient until you work on your emotional issues which cause you to attract them. Once you do that, they will begin to clear out of your life. You are of no use to them anymore.

[14]

Childhood Trauma & Chronic Lyme Disease

The Alice Miller books cited previously have demonstrated that childhood trauma can lead to emotional issues, and that emotional issues eventually lead to illness. The "Turning Gold into Lead" study mentioned in chapter 8 is a scientific study documenting the devastating effect of childhood trauma on people's health.

There are many types of trauma and many emotional patterns. I have spent a great deal of time discussing emotional issues here, which I am intimately familiar with. What is the relevance of these issues to chronic Lyme disease?

Chronic Lyme Patients Share Issues

I have found anecdotally that the emotional issues I'm familiar with are quite common among people with chronic

Lyme disease, but I never knew exactly why. It seemed like a coincidence, until I kept finding the same thing over and over.

Many Exposed to Lyme—Few Get Disease

I recalled a comment a doctor made to me in 2005. He said his testing indicated that about twenty-five percent of the general population has Lyme bacteria in their bodies. However, twenty-five percent of the population does not develop Lyme disease, even though they may have the bacteria in their bodies. I never knew why that was true. If a group of people are all exposed to the bacteria, then why do some get the disease and the rest do not? The gut flora issue related to lack of breastfeeding is a good candidate as a contributing factor, but what about the common emotional issues?

Many Exposed to Warfare—Few Get PTSD

Recently, I have been doing energy healing work in a program with veterans, many of whom have Post Traumatic Stress Disorder (PTSD). It turns out that the soldiers who get PTSD are typically the ones who had childhood trauma. Research confirms this as a causative factor. So here is another case in which a large group of people are exposed to a similar circumstance, warfare, but only some in the group acquire PTSD, while the rest do not.

Childhood Trauma Is the Link

I suspect the same is true for Lyme—while many people are exposed to Lyme bacteria, the only ones who actually develop Lyme disease are the ones who had some form of childhood trauma. The early trauma led to the emotional issues, which caused the stress that interfered with the nervous system and immune response. Therefore, the emotional issues of people with chronic Lyme disease are likely to be similar because childhood trauma is the common factor in their backgrounds.

Emotional Healing Is the Solution

While childhood trauma may have lain the foundation for the emotional issues that led to chronic Lyme disease, it is clear that the healing of these emotional issues can lead the way out.

[15]

How Did We Get into This Mess?

WHO CAN WE BLAME?

Alice Miller says that we have only one weapon against mental illness and that is to discover, through our emotions, the truth of the history of our own individual childhoods.[1]

CAN WE BLAME OUR PARENTS?

So if the way you were raised is what caused these early childhood traumas which led to emotional issues and illness, is it time to start pointing fingers? Even if you did, it wouldn't help. Did your parents do something wrong? No, they were just doing the best they could. They were raised the same way they raised you. It's all they knew. They thought they were doing the right thing. As Alice Miller demonstrates again and again in her books, these issues are

passed down generation to generation unconsciously—
nobody is aware it's happening. Childhood trauma is not
just about the effects of people who beat or severely abuse
their children. Trauma is far more common than previously
thought, as was shown in the scientific study "Turning Gold
into Lead" (see chapter 8).

CAN WE BLAME FATE?

So if it's not your parents' fault, can we at least blame
fate for giving us these parents? You can if you want. Personally, I believe we come into this life to learn soul lessons,
and we choose the parents who will wound us in the perfect
way to give us the issues we need in order to learn our life
lessons. If we choose our parents, how can we blame them?
You may not share these beliefs, but clearly these emotional
patterns exist, and we need to resolve them regardless of
how you think they came about. And blame won't help.

CAN WE BLAME THOSE WHO HAVE HURT US?

Well, can we at least blame the people who abused, betrayed, and abandoned us? No. We attracted them. They are
just doing what they do, learning their own lessons on their
own paths, and we attracted them into our path for our lessons. Actually, the lessons were mutual—you played a part
in their lessons as well. If you have adopted these types of
beliefs, life's mysteries can make more sense. It's not all
some tragic accident in which we are helpless victims. We
chose this path. It is for learning. However, if you have not
come to these beliefs, it still makes sense that emotional

issues underlie physical health, and that emotional healing is a wise course of action. It might be tempting to blame the people who have caused many of these problems in your life, but blame is a big issue in itself. It leads to chronic resentment and a victim complex.

YOU ARE NOT A VICTIM

The beauty of the spiritual view of things is that everything in your life comes back to you, which is empowering. There are no causes of your experience outside of yourself. But understanding this in a rational way is not enough. You still have to process your emotional issues. The good news in this is that you are not a helpless victim. If you work on your issues, you can alter your patterns, feel better, attract better partners, and heal your physical illness.

[16]

Expected Results of Emotional Healing

All the time that I was working on emotional healing, I did it with the intent of changing my life to make it better. I believed that resolving my issues would make them go away, and that my repeating patterns would stop. This would make me happier, attract better relationships, and recover my health.

Learning about the Cause of Issues

What I actually accomplished was a little different. First I learned a great deal about the issues I went through as an infant and how they affected my life. I was unaware of much of that before. It is quite helpful to learn about these things, because you may have habits which you have been beating yourself up over for years. When you know the emotional cause was something that happened to you as an infant, it allows you to stop blaming yourself. People often consider addiction to be a lack of willpower, when that couldn't be further from the truth. Blaming yourself for failure in dealing with it just adds a layer of shame and guilt on top of the issue, which strengthens its hold on you. If you have repeating patterns of being betrayed or abandoned, it can take a heavy toll on your self-esteem. If you discover the original cause as something that someone inadvertently did to you very early in life, then you can find some compassion for yourself.

YOUR PATTERNS DON'T ALL DISAPPEAR

Your emotional patterns don't magically vanish when you do emotional healing, but you don't react to them as much anymore. You can let yourself off the hook and stop berating yourself because of them. It wasn't your fault. It may not have been anyone's fault. You just reacted to it in an unfortunate but necessary way in order to survive. Having self-worth issues because someone betrayed you as an infant is like having a scar on your elbow because you fell off your bike as a kid. The effects of the wound are still there, but it's no big deal. It's just something that happened. You don't need to take it so personally. It wasn't really about you. The other person had his or her own stuff going on at the time.

So if all the issues didn't suddenly disappear, what did happen? First of all, some of the issues *did* disappear. For the ones that didn't, I found that I learned a lot about myself, which allowed me to have compassion for myself. A large portion of that reservoir of stuck energy from my emotional issues has been drained, so I find that I no longer react to many of the things that used to trigger me. I don't get upset as easily as I used to. Many things don't bother me at all anymore. My depression is gone. Some of my patterns have shifted, though not all. From a psychic point of view, my energy field has improved significantly. And, of course, the reason I started all this was because of health. My healing progressed to deeper levels, which led to a complete recovery from chronic Lyme disease.

FINDING SPACE AROUND YOUR ISSUES

Instead of making all the emotional issues and patterns disappear, what happens in healing is that you form space around them. They don't really bother you anymore. The reason you form space around these issues is partly because you have depleted the reservoir of stuck energy related to them, and partly because the issues themselves were a lie to begin with. Your perfect soul incarnates into a body, and you forget who you are and develop all kinds of beliefs that make you feel that you have little worth, when nothing could be further from the truth. So the patterns may still be there because you've had them for decades, but now, as you continue through these patterns, you kind of chuckle at them as they come up, *Oh, I still react to that situation. Isn't that funny.*

WHAT ISSUES?

I was surprised to find that one result of emotional healing was to develop space around my emotional issues. I don't take the events of my life so personally anymore. It's just stuff that happened. I went about trying to solve my issues and in the process, I got to a place where they weren't issues at all anymore.

[17]

Summary of Emotional Healing

- Childhood trauma is far more common than people think. It does not require abuse. It is the way the child perceives an event that matters.

- Emotional issues develop due to early childhood trauma that causes repeating behavior patterns.

- The body remembers everything. Physical symptoms are the body's way of indicating that an emotional wound has occurred, even if you can't remember it.

- Emotions are just energy that wants to move through our bodies. When emotions are suppressed or avoided the energy does not move through, and it gets stuck in our bodies.

- Continued suppression or avoidance of emotions causes the stuck energy to build up. This reservoir of stuck energy in our bodies hinders our life in many ways.

- The reservoir of stuck energy due to emotional issues, if not addressed, eventually manifests as illness.

- If the emotional issues underlying physical illness are deep enough, no amount of medication will resolve the physical problem until the underlying emotional issues are resolved.

- Dissipating the reservoir of stuck energy from emotional issues eliminates the underlying causes of physical illness. This facilitates physical healing.

- When an emotional issue is triggered, that issue is coming up for processing. Your body is an emotional energy dissipater. Consciously feeling the feelings that come up will process that energy out of your body.

- There are many emotional healing modalities to help process emotional issues.

RESOURCES

BOOKS

- *The Drama of the Gifted Child* - Alice Miller (explains how upbringing creates emotional patterns)
- *The Body Never Lies* - Alice Miller (explains how emotional patterns lead to chronic illness)
- *Heal Your Body A-Z* - Louise Hay (emotional causes of illness; listed by illness)
- *A New Earth, Awakening to Your Life's Purpose* - Eckhart Tolle (discusses many issues of the human emotional makeup)
- *Healing the Shame that Binds You* - John Bradshaw (explains more about the effects of upbringing)
- *For Your Own Good* - Alice Miller (documents examples of how upbringing creates emotional patterns)

WEBSITES

- Website on narcissism: **www.halcyon.com/jmashmun/npd/traits.html**
- Access Consciousness: **www.accessconsciousness.com**
- EFT: **www.emofree.com**
- Pranic Healing: **www.pranichealing.com**
- Radical Forgiveness: **www.radicalforgiveness.com**
- Release Technique: **www.releasetechnique.com**
- Theta Healing: **www.thetahealing.com**
- Byron Katie: **www.thework.com/en**
- Panache Desai: **www.panachedesai.com**

PRACTITIONERS

- **Bart Sharp** - Energy Healer in Austin, TX - specializes in emotional healing (www.bartsharp.com)

PART III

SPIRITUAL HEALING

[18]

My Story - 2015

I had been working night and day, researching and experimenting during my physical healing for ten years. Then I went into emotional healing with the same intensity—day and night—for three years (while continuing with the physical healing), and for the past year, 2015, I have been in what I call "spiritual healing." It involves learning the concept of nonresistance. This concept is typically discussed in spiritual circles. The comparable concept of surrender can be found in religious circles, though there is not much guidance on how to achieve it. It is only after thirteen years on this healing path that I evolved to learn this concept and how to use it. While it is a spiritual concept, it still pertains to emotional issues.

Working to Change My Life

Why did I work so hard on all this healing for thirteen years? I wanted to heal physically so I could feel better and get my life back. When I got into the emotional level of healing, I realized there were a lot of issues to heal there that I never even knew about, so all the stuff I had to heal was now expanding. Now I could change my emotional life for the better, and it would also help my physical healing. I am a hard worker. All my life, I have accomplished almost anything I set my mind to by working hard. I was a no-pain-no-gain type of guy. I like the concept because it gives me control over my life. I can always adjust how hard I work at anything, so if hard work is what brings results, then I have what it takes. I've been very successful in life by applying this principle. Every lesson I ever learned in my life seemed to have validated this principle. As I worked away at solving my health problems for the last thirteen years, I was working for that one future day when success was achieved, my health was recovered, and I could just be happy and live.

LIVING IN RESISTANCE

So in January 2015, as I was finishing up three years of emotional healing and not knowing what was to come next on my journey, I found myself at a retreat with a spiritual teacher named Panache Desai. One of his comments was, "Stop trying to change your life, and accept the life that you have. Trying to change your life is resistance to what is." Whoa! That was a jolt. That just blew up my whole model for living that I'd been using my entire life. All the work I had been doing to heal my life was for the purpose of changing it, so I was actually doing all that in resistance. In fact, the whole model of treating illness is by *fighting* it, which is again resistance. On top of that, I was not living in the present. I was putting off living until sometime in the future when all my health and emotional issues were better. Well, you can only live in the present moment. The past and future do not exist; they are just thoughts. If you are thinking about the future, then you are thinking that thought now instead of being present. This is a way of resisting the present moment, and if you're doing it, you are resisting life, because the present moment is the only place where life happens. I have been doing this all my life.

So I had just realized that something about my healing path the previous thirteen years had been misaligned. It was all done in resistance.

[19]

Resistance & Acceptance

RESISTANCE

Eckhart Tolle talks about resistance as an internal contraction. You close yourself off internally and remain in a state of negativity. Nothing is allowed in. If you take any action from this state, it will create more resistance. The universe will not assist you. However, if you yield internally and let go of the resistance, new doorways of consciousness are available to you and a new creative intelligence will support you. The universe becomes your ally. Friendly circumstances appear, coincidences happen, and people become helpful.[1]

There is a saying that "Your body can heal anything, but you have to get your mind out of the way first." What this means is that your body has an innate healing mechanism, and it's actually more powerful than you realize. But if you are constantly trying to get away from the condition you are in—illness—then you are in resistance to *what is*. What causes resistance? Judgment. You can be ill, you can feel sad, and you can be depressed, all without resistance—they are what they are. But when you judge those conditions as "bad", resistance begins. This causes suffering and leads to negative thinking and feeling. You want to avoid your physical illness, you want to avoid how you feel about it, and you want to avoid the negative thoughts and feelings that are created out of all this avoidance, because none of it feels good. As we saw in "Part II - Emotional Healing", if you are avoiding feeling emotions—typically ones that feel uncomfortable—then that causes the emotional energy to get stuck in your body, and it builds up as this keeps happening. This stuck energy works against your body's innate healing mechanism.

WANTING TO GET BETTER IS RESISTANCE

If you have been sick with chronic Lyme disease for a few years and you are not getting better, and you have thoughts that you might never get better, it can be devastating. The fear of never getting better can be overwhelming. The sadness you experience as you watch your life go by, knowing you can't do the things you used to do is painful.

You don't like where you are. You want to be someplace else. You are sick, and you want to get better. It's normal to feel this way, but this is resistance. It is resistance to your illness, how you feel in the present moment, and actually to life itself. Life is presenting itself as illness at the moment, so if you resist illness, you are resisting life. As you stay in resistance for years, it creates more resistance. Your thoughts and emotions about your situation are resistant. You don't like feeling bad. You complain. You go to doctors and they don't help, which makes you angry. You do more research and try new things, and it doesn't help, so you get frustrated. All of this feels bad, and you get tired of feeling bad. You are trying to avoid anything that feels bad, so all of this negative emotional energy is getting stuck in your body, instead of passing through.

Thoughts and emotions each contribute to the other, so this can create a downward spiral to a very dark place quickly. Repetitive thinking and feeling form beliefs, so if you form beliefs about never getting better, your body responds emotionally. Your body doesn't know the difference between reality and belief. It responds to either as if it were true. So now you have formed a repeating pattern of the vicious cycle of negative thinking and feeling which is creating negative beliefs, and this goes on day after day. You are in complete resistance to your illness, so all this emotional energy is getting stuck in your body.

This is a huge toxic load of stuck emotional energy on your body day in and day out, and it is accumulating.

THE ENERGY SITUATION

In Part II we discussed how the stuck energy of long-term emotional issues eventually manifests as illness. So you already had a reservoir of stuck energy in your body which caused your illness.

Now, you are creating a new reservoir of stuck energy due to this compounding resistance to your illness that you feel on a daily basis, year after year. This new reservoir is building on top of the one that already existed which caused your illness in the first place.

RESISTANCE BLOCKS HEALING

Can you imagine the effect all this toxic energy has on your body? Your body's innate healing mechanism was already trying to do its work in spite of interference from the original reservoir of stuck energy, and now you're piling on a lot more stuck emotional energy each day. Generating massive resistance to your body's healing efforts is the last thing you wanted to do, and you are probably unaware that you are even doing it. So now that you realize it, what are you supposed to do? Just stop thinking and feeling? Good luck with that. How about positive thinking? A well-intending person might suggest, "Hey, stop being so negative and maybe you'll feel better." Great! . . . problem solved. You might reply, "You try having the flu for eight f$%king years while your life is falling apart and tell me how positive you are, a$%hole." That's called Lyme rage. Add a parasite infestation which makes you irritable and angry all the time, and that poor guy will need a visit to the emergency room.

TYPICAL SPIRITUAL PRACTICES

Spiritual practices on issues like this tend to be in the nature of positive thinking, prayer, meditation, forgiveness, or gratitude. You've probably tried these. Maybe they helped some, but you're still stuck in this illness. In any case, positive thinking is not considered here, and prayer is up to you. I'll mention forgiveness and gratitude later, but there are two methods discussed here in regard to breaking down this massive resistance of thought and emotional energy you are generating on a daily basis. They are practical, effective, and cost nothing. Anyone can do them. They will change the course of your healing.

If this daily resistance you are creating is caused by negative thoughts and feelings, then there are two ways to break it down. The next chapter will present a method of nonresistance using your feelings. You will learn how to use all these negative feelings to actually heal yourself. The following chapter will present a method of nonresistance using your thoughts.

ACCEPTANCE

A discussion of nonresistance automatically brings to mind the related concept of acceptance. When you mention the word "acceptance," some people get turned off. They think if you accept a situation that you are just giving up, and you will be stuck with the situation you want to change. This is a weak, passive type of acceptance. The type of acceptance we are working with in this book might be called "allowance." Allowance is a form of acceptance when you stand firmly in your power and allow a situation to be what it is, without resistance. This is a strong, active type of acceptance. Allowance simply means that you accept the fact that a situation exists, not that you have a favorable inclination to the situation itself.

The concept being conveyed in this book with nonresistance is that you need to be in a neutral place in order to bring about change in a situation. Resistance to a situation just creates more resistance, and so makes change difficult. What you resist persists. The discussion of nonresistance in this book will always be using the "allowance" type of acceptance. You observe a situation without judgment. You are neither acquiescing nor fighting it.

[20]

Nonresistance Method Using Feelings

PANACHE DESAI'S WORK

The method of nonresistance presented in this chapter is based on the work of Panache Desai. Panache is a spiritual teacher, among other titles. He is known as a vibrational transformation specialist for his energetic abilities. I've studied his work in retreats and through online programs throughout 2015. I have taken part in several of his ten-day and twenty-one-day energetic programs which clear vibrational density (stuck emotional energy), and I've read his book *Discovering Your Soul Signature*.[1]

EMOTIONS—ENERGY IN MOTION

This is a short summary of Panache Desai's teachings in regard to emotions and nonresistance. He teaches that emotions are just energy which is trying to run through us.

We have no control over emotions. Situations trigger them. They have no particular meaning. It is pointless to judge emotions. They are neither good nor bad, but some emotions can be painful. When we judge painful emotions as "bad," we tend to suppress them or try to avoid them. Avoiding these emotions causes the emotional energy to get stuck in our bodies, instead of running through us. Panache calls this stuck energy *vibrational density*, and we have built up quite a bit of it over the course of our lives. (Note that his term "vibrational density" is the same concept as "stuck energy" that was used in "Part II - Emotional Healing.") Children haven't learned how to avoid their emotions, so they just process feelings as they come. Children will cry when sad, throw a tantrum when angry, or scream in terror when afraid, and then they are fine five minutes later after letting all the energy run through their bodies. It is only when parents teach children that it isn't appropriate to act out or cry that they learn to suppress emotions.

RESISTANCE TO OUR EMOTIONS

As we get older, we don't like painful emotions. We resist pain, so we find ways to suppress these feelings or avoid them. We find distractions like drinking, smoking, eating, having sex, etc. to avoid feeling our emotions. If you are avoiding an emotion, then you are in resistance to it which causes the energy to get stuck in your body. This creates vibrational density; however, when we feel our emotions consciously, the energy runs through us and processes out of our bodies. If we just felt all our feelings like children, then we wouldn't create any vibrational density at all. The density which has built up in our bodies is what blocks our energy in all areas of our lives, including physical healing.

The best way to let go of resistance is to just feel your feelings consciously, and to process vibrational density out of your body.

FEELING CONSCIOUSLY

To feel your feelings consciously means to actively focus on the sensations in your body, and the location where you feel them, without judging them as good or bad. You don't need to think about the story, or judge yourself for having the feeling. Just focus on feeling the sensation in your body, like a detached observer. If you keep doing this, the emotional energy will run through your body and process out of you. Panache uses the analogy of sailing in a boat at sea. If there is a storm coming with large waves, you would typically want to sail in the opposite direction to avoid the storm. In the case of emotions, however, he says you should turn your boat into the storm. It may seem counterintuitive, but sailing into the storm is the way through. In regard to emotions, this means to feel everything there is to feel about the situation. In doing this, you are processing energies out of your body that you were previously in resistance to. Now you are in nonresistance to your emotions. And as feelings occur in the present moment, then you are in non resistance to the present moment, and to life.

Feeling Unconsciously

Feeling your emotions consciously can be tricky when you are triggered by a real life event. If you become very angry at someone, you may get so lost in the anger that you cannot consciously focus on the sensations in your body. If you are projecting your anger outwardly at a person in blame, then you are feeling your emotions *unconsciously*, or without awareness of what you are feeling. This creates more vibrational density instead of dismantling it, so you have to be prepared to maintain composure when you get triggered and just feel the emotions in your own body. This is taking responsibility for your internal state, because it really has nothing to do with anyone else. External events may seem like they cause emotions, but they don't. They just trigger something that is already inside you. The same external event that triggers you one day may not trigger you at all on another day, because your internal state is different. Taking responsibility for your internal state means choosing not to react and just observe the sensation as the energy runs through your body.

So these are some of the teachings of Panache Desai in regard to emotions and nonresistance that I have absorbed over the last year. The following describes how to apply this method to your emotions in chronic Lyme disease, so you can heal yourself.

Applying this Nonresistance Method to Chronic Lyme Disease

Let's be clear about what we are not resisting. Nonresistance, in this case, means not resisting whatever emotions are coming up for you in the present moment.

We are not trying to be in nonresistance to illness. That is a mental concept, and how you feel about that concept will change from day to day due to your internal state. Life happens only in the present moment. As we are in nonresistance to the emotions that come up in each moment, we are no longer resisting the ever-changing flow of life, or trying to control it. If life happens in the present moment, then your healing happens in the present moment as well.

Resistance to Emotions in Illness

As we discussed in the last chapter, you don't like where you are, and you want to be someplace else. You are sick, and you want to get better. You are resisting your physical illness, how you feel emotionally about it, and actually life itself. Life is presenting itself as illness at the moment, so if you resist it, you are resisting life.

The more you want to get better, and the more it doesn't happen, the greater your resistance becomes to your present state. Resistance creates more resistance. You have formed a repeating pattern of the vicious cycle of negative thinking and feeling which is creating negative beliefs, and this goes on day after day, year after year. You are in complete resistance to your illness, so all this emotional energy is getting stuck in your body.

This is a huge toxic load on your body, and it is accumulating daily. When you understand what effect emotions have on your health, and you realize what emotions you are experiencing every day with your illness, you can see that this is not helping you. You are already feeling these emotions. It's just that you have been feeling them unconsciously in resistance, which builds vibrational density. Your body holds this density which blocks your healing.

Panache's technique is a way of feeling the emotions in nonresistance, which breaks down vibrational density and facilitates your healing. It doesn't matter whether your emotions are pleasant or unpleasant; it only matters whether you resist them or allow them as they are. It seems counterintuitive to embrace your feelings of misery when all you want to do is run away from them, but when you break down this vibrational density that you create every day, you are clearing the path for the body's innate healing mechanism to proceed without interference. You are getting your mind out of the way, so to speak.

"Part II - Emotional Healing" discussed working on the past emotional issues you built up all your life, which caused your illness. In this "Part III - Spiritual Healing," we are now talking about the present emotional issues you are creating daily through resistance to your present state.

In chronic Lyme, you've taken that normal process of building vibrational density over the course of your life and stepped on the accelerator, pushing it into overdrive, and you're now doing this 24/7. I didn't start to feel better for eight years when I was sick, so you can imagine what kind of negative thoughts and emotions I was generating. I've been depressed most of my adult life, and being sick for many years didn't exactly improve that. Your body is trying to heal, but your thoughts and emotions are working overtime to snuff out those efforts. We are creating massive resistance, yet we remain unaware that we are doing it.

RESISTANCE HARMS YOUR HEALTH

As humans, we evaluate things. On a daily basis, you evaluate whether your health is getting better or worse. If it's not getting better, then you believe you are headed in the wrong direction, and this makes you feel bad. This type of thinking is natural, yet it is causing harm to your health.

People often focus only on physical healing and never even consider that their emotions have anything to do with it, but we've established in Part II how important emotions are to your physical health. That reservoir of vibrational density that you built up during your life caused your illness, and now you're adding to it—big time. The suffering you feel, because you resist the physical and emotional discomfort of illness, is the most natural reaction that any person could have, but this resistance is interfering with your healing.

So what can you do?

Stop the resistance.

How to Stop the Resistance

You don't need to try to avoid the vicious cycle of negative thinking and feeling. Avoiding all that would be more resistance, plus, it's virtually impossible. For starters, accept that you are feeling miserable and your thinking is really negative, and at this moment, you feel like life is hopeless. You have every right to feel that way; anyone would, so accepting that these feelings exist is just acknowledging reality. Now, momentarily, you are no longer resisting your thoughts and emotions. This is your first step. Nonresistance is the key to moving forward. You don't have to feel good to be in nonresistance. You just have to allow the present moment to be what it is, even if it feels miserable. You feel your feelings without judging them or trying to avoid them. You just observe.

Example of Nonresistance Method

Now that you aren't judging your feelings in the present moment, what do you do with them? Keep feeling them. Sit with them until you don't feel them anymore.

Let's run through how to use this non-resistance method with some examples of different emotions that typically come up.

Feeling Hopeless

When you've been sick for a few years, and you begin to realize your illness is just not getting better, no matter what you do, or how many doctors you see, how does that make you feel? Where do you feel that in your body? In your gut?

Then focus on that feeling in your gut and just sit with the physical sensations of it without judging it.

Think thoughts that stir up those feelings. If you're not getting better, you've tried everything, you've read a lot of books, you're spending too much money, and you're too tired to fight anymore, how does that make you feel? Where do you go from here? Are you really just going to be sick for the rest of your life? Feel the hopelessness in your gut that has been building for years. You've been trying to hold back the despair for so long and soldier on, but now it's time to just allow it to come forth without judging it. Let it out. Continue to just feel it in your gut until you don't feel it anymore. Make sure you focus on the physical sensation in your gut. Don't be afraid. You're already feeling this stuff, but now you're doing it in a way that heals you. Is this painful? Yeah. But so is life the way it is now anyway.

NOTE ON FEELING THE SENSATIONS IN YOUR BODY

The part of this method about feeling emotions as a sensation in your body is critical. There is a loop where negative thoughts cause negative emotions, and those emotions then feed back into more negative thoughts. This loop keeps going around in a vicious cycle. The thoughts are connected to the emotions. However, when you feel a negative emotion only as a physical sensation in your body, you disconnect the thought from the emotion and you ground the cycle in your body. The emotion can then no longer feed back into the loop of negative thinking. The vicious cycle has been broken. At this point, the emotional energy is flowing only one way—out of your body.

FEELING SAD

Are you sad because you see life going by? You have only so much time on this planet, and it's going by, and you're not even getting better. People you know are enjoying their lives, but you live in a different world now. It's like there's a plate glass window separating your world from theirs, and you're on the outside looking in. Did you have a fun life before the illness and now it's all gone? Did you like outdoor activities or traveling in the past, but now you can't do them anymore? Did you have a good marriage, but it ended when you got sick because you were miserable all the time? Where do you feel that in your body? Focus on that. Just be with the feelings in your body without judging them. Feel the heartbreak. Let the dam burst. Cry it out.

Think thoughts that stir up those feelings. Look at some old photos of your trips, or your relationship. This triggers the vibrational density stored in your body to make more of it come up, so you can feel it and then process it out. The more you consciously feel these feelings, the more you burn off the density. Stay with the feeling in the body as long as it lasts. It might take twenty minutes or more.

You know that crying has made you feel better when you've been sad in the past. You stopped the resistance to the sadness and just felt it, so it released. This process of feeling all your feelings is doing the same thing for all the emotions.

You are clearing the stuck energy, or vibrational density, that you've been building up in your body every day, which is blocking your path to healing. Before you were just clogging it up. It's important to really focus on the sensations in your body. If you focus on the story too much, this can pull you back into your mind where you lose focus on your body.

Once you process a lot of the pain out of your body, you will be able to remember the memories and look at the old photos without feeling pain. The photos don't cause the pain. They just trigger the stuck energy of that pain that's already inside of you, that you never processed before. Now you're processing it out. When it's gone, the photos can't trigger you anymore, because there is no energy in there to get triggered. If you understand the mechanics of this process, you can see it's not really so personal. When you focus on a sensation in your body, you separate it from the thought. The thoughts and feelings together cause intense pain, but when you disconnect the two, the pain becomes more manageable. This can give you more courage to really go for it. This is tough at first, but after you process a bunch of the density out of you it becomes easier, and you can handle more at one time.

FEELING LIKE A VICTIM

Do you feel like a victim of fate, illness, spirochetes, parasites, your body, God (one of my personal favorites)? Are you powerless to change your circumstances? Do you believe it's absolutely impossible to get rid of parasites and there's nothing you can ever do (I've been there)? Okay, so you're a victim. It's pretty tough to be sick every day for years and not feel like a victim. But many will say, "Pull yourself together. If you believe you are a victim, then you are one." While there may be some truth to that in regard to the effects of belief, what we are dealing with here are the effects of your feelings. Those feelings are coming up now and they need to be addressed.

We don't need to judge feelings, just process them. So if you are arguing with yourself about how you *shouldn't* be a victim, then you've gotten lost in your mind. Focus on the feelings in the body. If the feelings of powerlessness and being a victim are coming up now, then just feel them. Where in your body do you feel them? Focus on the sensation of that, wherever you feel it in your body. Consciously wallow in the victimhood to keep it flowing, and keep feeling it in the body until it's gone. When it comes back tomorrow, feel it some more. You are not resisting or fighting anything here. You're just feeling the feelings in your body—that magical dissipater of the stuck emotional energy that blocks your life. If you have a belief that you are a victim, and you keep attracting situations which make you feel like a victim—which is what repeating patterns do—the best way out of it is to process out all of the victim energy inside of you which is what we are doing here.

This may seem contrary to teachings that we should not be victims. People keep telling themselves, *I am not a victim. I am not a victim.* But that is just avoiding what you really feel. If at that moment you feel like a victim, then process that emotion out by feeling it.

If you wallow in victimhood "unconsciously", by complaining and feeling sorry for yourself, you are creating vibrational density. If you wallow in victimhood "consciously", by just focusing on the sensation it causes in your body, you are dissipating vibrational density.

In regard to victimization, we often use it to cover up our own issues that we are afraid to look at. It's easier to blame someone or something for causing our problems rather than to accept that they are just our own issues. It helps you maintain a little dignity, but if you want to resolve your issues, you need to forget about dignity. Besides, when you do this process and separate the feelings from the thoughts, you don't take your issues so personally anymore. So there's no need to use victimization as a fig leaf anymore.

NOTE ON JUDGING YOUR EMOTIONS

It's important to note that you don't argue with yourself in order to logically justify your feelings like, *I shouldn't be angry at so-and-so over this little thing. Anger doesn't solve anything. I shouldn't be afraid of that. Being a victim is bad, so I'll just be strong.* Feelings don't need to be judged, just felt. Whatever comes up in the present moment is felt and processed whether it is rational or not, or whether you like it or not. If you are enraged over some perceived slight that you've only imagined, that's okay. Let it out. Your body has brought the feeling up for processing, so go with it. If you are arguing with what comes up in the present moment, then you are in your head. You are not only judging the emotion, but judging yourself for having it. That is just more resistance. Feelings have no meaning. They are just energy wanting to run through, so let them.

FEELING ANGER

Are you angry that a stupid insect caused you all this trouble? Are you angry at life? Are you angry at God for allowing this? What is the point of this exactly? Why are other people spared this trial, but you have to go through it? Perhaps your friends and loved ones don't want to be around you anymore. You know you're not a lot of fun anymore, but you were there for them when they were down. This isn't fair. Where do you feel the anger in your body? Focus on that sensation and feel the anger without judging it. How does the physical sensation of anger feel compared to sadness? Anger is a charged energy that runs through your body like an electrical current.

NOTE ON EXPRESSING EMOTIONS TO OTHERS

It is important to note here that we are talking about *feeling* emotions in your body, not *expressing* them to other people. Yelling at another person to express anger is not what is recommended here—that is not taking responsibility for your internal state. Sometimes you may need to express your emotions to another, and how you do that is your choice, but this process is about how you run the emotional energy through your own body in order to burn it off. If you need to get a big stick and beat the crap out of some pillows, or scream into a pillow, go ahead. Feel the feelings and process the energy. Nonresistance does not imply peace and serenity. It implies being with whatever is happening in the moment without resisting it. If what is happening in the moment is rage, then nonresistance means feeling that rage without judging it. Let it rip.

FEELING FEAR

Are you seeing the best doctors, doing hours of research daily, and paying a lot of money for your treatment, and you still aren't getting any better? Are you terrified that not only is your life going down, but your treatment is draining the precious resources your family needs to live on? Are you afraid you'll lose your job because you take too many sick days, and your attitude is not so pleasant anymore? Is your partner looking to end your relationship? Are you going to be sick for the rest of your life? If you are alone and unemployed, how will you survive? Where do you feel that in your body? Just focus on that sensation in your body and sit with it without judging it. Keep feeling the fear until it dissipates. It may take a while. When you reach a point where thinking about the issue no longer stirs up the feeling of fear, you're done . . . for today anyway. Can you tell the difference between the physical sensations of fear and anger?

FEELING GUILT

Do you feel guilty because you no longer want to do many activities with your kids? Are you irritable and snap at your family too often? Do you realize that you're not being the parent you wanted to be? Are you no longer able to be a good partner to your spouse? Are expensive treatments draining family resources, and you're not getting better? Do you feel guilty because all you want to do is lie on the couch all day in your pajamas and watch TV? You don't really look sick, and you know what people are thinking. Where do you feel the guilt in your body? Focus on the sensation of that. Keep feeling it until it's gone. Know that as you feel the sensation in your body consciously, you are dissipating the energy that blocks your healing. Allow the feelings to come. Don't suppress the guilt. Feeling it is how you get rid of it.

FEELING LONG-TERM EMOTIONAL ISSUES

This method has been focused on the new emotional issues you create daily due to resistance to your illness. This is in addition to the vibrational density from your long-term issues which caused your illness in the first place as discussed in Part II.

However, I suspect that as you work on these more recent emotional issues, you are also working on your long-term issues simultaneously. For instance, in the anger example above, the issue of abandonment—friends not wanting to be around you—came up which is a long-term emotional pattern. When you work on sadness, if you have a pattern where sadness spirals into depression, then you are tapping into a long-term issue. This is the work that was discussed in "Part II - Emotional Healing" where you can directly heal the cause of your illness by working on long-term issues. These patterns didn't take a break just because you got sick. In fact, the long-term emotional patterns you have had all your life have probably kicked into overdrive in your illness. So they are intermingled with the current emotions you are experiencing which create resistance.

This method was originally meant to break down your current resistance caused by feeling your emotions unconsciously on a daily basis, which was interfering with your body's innate healing ability. That, in itself, would be a big improvement in your healing process. However, when you also start breaking down the reservoir of stuck energy, or vibrational density, of your long-term emotional issues, which are what caused your illness, you are directly healing the underlying cause of your illness. You are killing two birds with one stone, and it hasn't cost you a dime.

PRACTICE

I would suggest that as you start doing this practice of feeling your feelings that you do it when you are in a decent mood and in a safe place. That way you can pick an issue, work on it, and let the emotions flow consciously without affecting anyone else. If you wait until you are triggered by six simultaneous real life events while surrounded by a group of people, and you're feeling overwhelmed, you may be feeling your emotions unconsciously and will be unable to practice this. After some amount of practice, you will develop proficiency at this, and then you will be prepared to handle real situations when you get triggered. When those happen, you need to be present enough to step back from the situation and just observe yourself while you feel the emotions running through your body.

Remember that when you feel your feelings unconsciously, judge them, complain about them, or try to avoid them, you are in resistance and adding to your vibrational density. When you feel your feelings consciously in your body, without judgment, allowing them to flow through while you observe them, you are reducing your vibrational density and healing yourself.

There is no harm in bringing up and feeling painful feelings. They're already there anyway. In fact, there is a huge benefit to bringing them up, because you are processing that emotional energy out of your body. As Rumi, the thirteenth-century Persian poet and Sufi master said, "The wound is the place where the light enters you."[2] So engage the suffering; that's where you'll find the healing. Turn the boat into the storm. But do it *consciously*. There is fear of painful emotions, but when you separate the physical sensation from the story of the emotion with this method, you'll find the pain is easier to tolerate.

Using this method is like doing an herbal cleanse for a week to detoxify your body. You know you might feel some ill effects along the way, but you accept it because you know there is a health benefit at the end. I use this method on a regular basis, and I feel like I am letting emotional toxins drain out of my body.

FUTURE OUTLOOK

Using this method will be a tough slog at first, so go easy on yourself. The process really picks up momentum after a while. The more stuck energy you process out, the better you feel, the more confidence you have that you're improving, and the more you want to go after deeper issues to process. But not at first. That's the slowest, hardest place in the process. So stick with it. It may seem like there is no end to the misery for a while, but there is. After doing a lot of this work, and crying a lot, you can go back and think of some memories and look at some photos, and you'll find you don't feel the pain anymore. It's not there anymore because you burned off all the energy of the pain that was inside you. That's when you know you are healing yourself. You're beginning to see results—a taste of success! You haven't burned off all the vibrational density in your body from your entire lifetime on any given issue, but you've burned off all the energy that was *available* for processing now. You'll have to do more on it another time when it comes up again. Some event, person, song, or memory will trigger you again someday, and you'll feel that pain again. When that happens, it's not a setback. We often think we are back at square one when this happens, because an issue we thought we had resolved has come back. It's not true. It's just that more of that energy deep inside you has shaken loose and is ready to come up and be processed out. So go through this process again. That's how it works. You can't get all the energy at one time.

Emotional energy comes up for processing when it's ready. It comes to the surface, you get triggered and you burn it off. Later, when more comes up, you burn off more. You start to work the give-and-take process of healing with your body. You learn to be patient and wait for your body.

Your body is in charge of this process. It will bring up the energy that you most need to burn off when it is available. Emotional healing is a lifetime process, so get in the habit of doing this over the long haul, and it will serve you well.

When you run out of current emotions to process, you can start dredging up old memories from your life that cause you pain. Do the same with those and just consciously feel the emotions that come up. I've completed this process with the memories, and I'm now searching for more issues to process. The farther you get in this process, the more peace you feel in your life.

I've heard of many techniques you can use to make unwanted feelings go away, but this one is the simplest, and works the best. If you don't like what you are feeling, just keep feeling it. Not only does it solve the problem by processing the emotion, but it makes it less likely the feeling will return again in the future because you are burning off the energy of it. If you avoid feeling the emotion, you can be sure it will return.

Recent Experiences

Recently, I was out at the store and started to feel bad emotionally for no reason. I was able to watch my train of thoughts in real time as the feeling came up. The thoughts went something like this: *I shouldn't be feeling like this. I don't like feeling like this. How can I change it? I was feeling good a little while ago. How do I get back to that? Is there a technique I can use to change this? Why did this happen? Did I do something wrong?* At that moment, I realized I was in resistance to what was happening, and remembered the best thing to do was to just keep feeling the feelings. So I did. I don't remember what happened after that because it didn't bother me anymore. That was easy. The easiest way out of the problem is through it. It's interesting when you get a glimpse of your thoughts. In that situation, my thoughts were in curiosity at first, but then started to trend negative. Be careful of asking "why" questions. Your mind will come up with some answer, and it might cause a negative emotion. My questions at the end were starting to begin a negative thinking loop which would lead to negative emotions. But even a negative thinking loop is no problem if you just feel your feelings with this method. It will stop the loop dead in its tracks.

While finishing this book, I started to ponder all the issues involved in publishing it. The issues are overwhelming and the learning curve was steep, so I would go into overwhelm when thinking about them. I could stop and take a break which would help, but the problem would be there when I came back to it. That was just avoidance. The overwhelm isn't caused by the situation. It's caused by how I handle it, which is a long-term emotional pattern. So whenever the overwhelm came up, I sat with it and felt it consciously in my gut, just letting it run out of me. This is easy.

SUMMARY

If you are going through this process to heal yourself, you are very courageous, and you're thinking outside of the box. You are no longer avoiding your fate. You are facing it, taking it head on, and doing the best thing you can possibly do to heal yourself. Healing is an inside job. A doctor can't do it all for you. You have the tools now, and you're developing the confidence. The tide has begun to turn. You are developing your power and you know it. The best part is that this process starts to get easier. Eventually, you start looking for things that trigger you so you can process more emotional energy.

Well, this is a huge turnaround in your healing process. Your physical healing will begin to move forward as you work on clearing your emotional density, but there will still be a challenging road ahead. I had several health crises after I began emotional healing. They seemed like setbacks to me, but they were actually breakthroughs. My physical health was jumping to a higher level as a result of the emotional healing, but it didn't happen overnight.

Consider, also, that as you go through this process of consciously feeling your feelings, you begin to lose the fear of feeling. You are no longer running away from your feelings. Some feelings are still painful, but that's no big deal anymore. You can handle it. Consciously feeling your feelings in your body also keeps you in the present moment.

If you learned to shut down your feelings as a child, then this practice is the way back to learning how to feel again. It's okay to feel now. There's no way back to living without feeling.

Nonresistance Method Using Thoughts

THEME OF ABRAHAM BOOK

There is a book that shares a great deal of wisdom on the need to come to a place of nonresistance in order to move forward in life, and it presents another method for doing this using thoughts. The book, *The Astonishing Power of Emotions*, by Esther and Jerry Hicks, presents the teachings of Abraham, a group of nonphysical entities whose messages are translated by Esther Hicks. Given that thoughts affect feelings, improved thoughts lead to improved feelings. The main concept of this book is that there is a flow of life, represented as a stream, with you on it in a rowboat. You can either go upstream against the flow, or downstream with the flow. The way to tell which way you are going is by how you feel at any given moment. If you feel stressed, you are going upstream; you are not aligned with your soul. If you feel at peace, you are going downstream; you are aligned with your soul. The interesting part of this concept is that Abraham states that everything you want is downstream. That means that if you are working hard toward a goal, then you are going upstream, and this is not what you want. The nonresistance method presented by Abraham is to modify your thoughts little by little until they become more positive, so that you feel better. Feeling better means you have come to a place of nonresistance. The way to describe this process of coming to nonresistance, with the metaphor of the rowboat, is that you just let go of the oars. When you stop paddling upstream, the current will gently turn your boat back downstream, where you can then flow effortlessly toward what you want.[1]

WHY NONRESISTANCE IS ESSENTIAL

The need to come into nonresistance is the same in this book as it was with the method from the last chapter. In fact, the Abraham book does a great job of explaining why nonresistance is the best way forward, as seen in the book's many case studies of real-life situations. Hard work and struggle are not the way. So again, if you are a no-pain-no-gain type of person, this is a rebuke. If you are fighting anything, then you are in resistance, and this is not the way to move forward.

Abraham talks about what it takes to move to a place of health from a place of illness. If the place of health will make you feel good, and right now you feel bad, then you are not moving toward your goal, because if you feel bad, you are moving upstream. If you want to move toward your goal, he says, "You have to feel good now, no matter what the conditions are, or the conditions cannot improve. You must make peace, so to speak, with where you are to allow yourself to move to a place you would rather be."[2] In other words, it is not the conditions that are important. The most important thing is whether or not you are in resistance to the conditions.

RESISTANCE BLOCKS PROGRESS

To continue to resist and complain about where you are will prevent improvement in your condition. You are paddling upstream. Making peace with where you are is nonresistance—letting go of the oars. Only then can you turn around and go downstream—forward toward what you want. You don't have to celebrate illness. You simply have to accept the fact that it is there. It is just reality.

MODIFYING THOUGHTS—CASE STUDIES

The book demonstrates how to use its method of modifying your thoughts in several case studies of real life situations. The first case study is of a person who has just received a diagnosis of illness and is worried. In this situation, a person would typically seek out a second opinion and then find doctors, treatments, and protocols which could help. It would typically be a time of frantic searching and trying to find a solution (see chapter 2 for my frantic search over the course of many years). However, Abraham's guidance in this situation is that the only thing you need to consider at that moment, right after diagnosis, is whether or not you are pointed upstream or downstream.[3] In other words, are you in resistance or nonresistance? That is more important than anything, because if you take action from a place of resistance, you will just create more resistance (as I did for thirteen years). If you fight illness, you create more illness. What you resist persists. Solutions are only available when you are in nonresistance. So how do you find out if you are moving upstream or downstream? By how you feel. If you are stressed, you're moving upstream. If you are peaceful, you're moving downstream.

A Different Perspective

Abraham says that the Law of Attraction's response to resistance is disease. It's response to nonresistance is well-being.[4]

This book provides another method of coming into nonresistance. It is well worth reading, regardless of whether or not you use this method. The book provides a great deal of wisdom, especially on the reasons why we need to come into nonresistance. All the case studies contain wisdom that will help you, not just the ones relating to illness.

[22]

Summary of the Two Nonresistance Methods

The nonresistance methods of Panache Desai and Abraham, described in the previous two chapters, provide a way of getting to a point where you are in nonresistance with your thoughts and feelings in each present moment. That is a place of neutrality from which you can move forward. One method works on feelings, the other on thoughts. Thoughts affect emotions and emotions affect thoughts, so either method will impact both thoughts and feelings.

That the rowboat metaphors of each method seem a bit conflicting is not significant. If you study both methods in depth, they are quite compatible. One just works with emotions and the other with thoughts. There are some subtle differences, but they are both making the same point about the need to come into nonresistance, and each offers a practical way to do that.

Personally, I prefer the method of feeling emotions. When emotions are running high, I find it hard to modify my thoughts in order to feel better. At these times, I find it more direct to just focus on letting the feelings run through. It is simple and direct. Plus, I've spent too much time in my head during my life. Now I find it more rewarding to work with feelings. I also like the idea of dissipating the reservoir of vibrational density with the method of feeling my emotions. Nonetheless, after emotions return to a more neutral place, I sometimes like to work on my thoughts. Everyone is different, however. In the end, it comes down to finding a method that works for you. Try them and see.

[23]

My Experience with Resistance

MEDICINE IS A RESISTANT PARADIGM

Consider that the typical way that medicine, conventional or alternative, modern or ancient, deals with illness is to fight it, overcome it, heal it or kill it. This is all resistance. Certainly, alternative medicine has more modalities that are in alignment with nature and could be considered more nonresistant; however, there are still modalities, such as antibacterial herbs, which kill things. The moment you enter the realm of medicine, you are in a resistant paradigm, and all your thoughts related to the application of medical treatments are resistant ones.

Take parasites, for example. I've spent fourteen years trying to kill them with every method known to mankind, all the while being frustrated about the whole situation. Then I worked on clearing the emotional issues related to parasites. This is better, but still resistant. What's left? Non-resistance. Parasites love the energy of irritation and anger. If you hate them, they love it; you can feel them getting stirred up when you have those feelings. Is resistance the best way to heal this problem? Is healing itself resistance? Is this a problem? Maybe if you sent love to parasites, they wouldn't be able to stand the high vibration of love and would have to leave? Maybe you can ask them to leave your body. I think this works, but your consciousness has to be at a high enough level. The parasites are there for some beneficial reason, as is the illness. They are serving some purpose. I'm not sure healing illness needs to be all about killing things.

LEARNING TO LIVE WITH PARASITES

I came upon the Abraham book (see chapter 21) in 2013. That was my first encounter with the concept of nonresistance. I was most of the way through my healing path at that point, though I was still dealing with parasites. I was able to apply the nonresistance concept to parasite treatment. I learned how to manage the parasites through diet and herbal treatments, and then I just decided to live with them without trying to get rid of them. I just accepted that health issues are part of life. The funny thing is that once you do this, issues begin to fall away, and often you don't even notice they're gone. As I reach the point now where the parasites are leaving completely, it is not that big of a deal, yet there was a time when they ruled my body, my emotions, and my life. I desperately fought to kill them with harsh treatments. The parasites were so impossible to eliminate that I used to take comfort in the thought that at least my death would one day terminate them.

I Was Always in Resistance

It was only in 2015 that I came upon Panache Desai's work with nonresistance. It came late on my healing path, but it expanded my understanding of this concept, which is helpful in other areas of my life, beyond physical health. There is something profound about processing your deepest, darkest, most painful emotions without judgment. You're jumping into the rabbit hole, and even though you don't know where it will come out, you know it's the right way to go. It's actually the only way to go. When you come out the other end, maybe the next step is to jump into a new rabbit hole, but that's okay. You know you're going the right way. Your soul has brought you on this journey for some reason, and you have to go along or you won't make it to the next level of the journey.

Prolonging My Illness

I can now see, very late in my healing journey, that I did not use nonresistance during my healing from chronic Lyme disease. Intuitives often told me that I was prolonging my own illness with all the suffering and resistance, but I didn't know what to do about it. How do you stop suffering? I just hadn't evolved to the place where I could learn nonresistance yet. For thirteen years, all of my physical

234 | *Robert Groleau*

healing occurred while my thoughts and emotions were in constant resistance to healing, and actually to life itself.

Fearing the Worst Possible Outcome

I had a big emotional pattern of fearing the worst possible outcome. In chapter 2, the episodes of: 2009 involving my gallbladder, 2010 with the return of Lyme symptoms, 2012 with parasites, and 2013 with the intestinal infection (and countless others not mentioned), all involved my having a severe bout of fearing the worst possible outcome, even though the outcome was unknown at the time. That is very hard on the healing process that your body is trying to maintain, not to mention the nervous system. The body is doing its healing work, and it then gets overwhelmed with all this toxic emotional energy that you're creating.

Saying No to Life

Resistance is about saying the word no—no to healing, no to your body which isn't working the way you want, and no to life. If you research the emotional issues underlying chronic illness, you will find "refusal to change, fear of the future,[1] and resistance to understand the messages."[2]

Do you have a secret desire to check out of life? Perhaps one purpose of illness is to force you to declare whether you're in or out. I had been in resistance to life all my life. Having a severe illness was a way to check out—it was the culmination of all my years of resistance. Life was often painful, so I never really committed to being here. This illness made me decide if I wanted to start saying yes to life.

That was scary. I thought, *Does this mean I have to accept all the painful stuff that happens? I don't really want to do that. I've kind of had enough of that.* Well, yes, you *do* have to accept all that, but it's in the accepting, or not resisting, that life gets easier. Who would have thought that surrender is the way to win the battle? So if you decide you want to say yes to life now, you'll have to do it within the confines of illness . . . life has upped the ante.

GUIDANCE

As for "resistance to understand the messages," well, there is a purpose to all this. The universe is on your side. It is conspiring to bring you what you desire. If you are not aware of this, it might seem impossible to believe, given what you are going through. But if your life's lessons were to overcome self-worth issues, this path would accomplish that by dragging you through all the muck of physical and then emotional healing. It can be difficult to see the purpose in it all. The lessons in the Earth school tend to be quite challenging. How steep your learning path is depends on what goal your soul chose for this life, and where you started from.

What *do* you really desire? That's what your soul chose before coming here. Things happen in their right time. This doesn't mean it is all pleasant. It's just that the universe is taking you through your lessons so you can have what you ultimately want. However, if you are not listening to the messages that guide you through your lessons, you'll get bogged down in resistance to the misery. It's hard to hear the messages when you're in resistance. It's nice to have accepted the concept that the universe is on your side, but I have to say that I found I was on a guided healing path long before I came to that understanding. My journey through Lyme disease was a rough one, but every time I hit a brick wall and thought I was done for, some treatment would bail me out—I never stopped searching. I didn't know why that was happening to me, but it happened enough times that I recognized it. It still took fourteen years, but there was help along the way. Are you getting your messages? Are you listening? Complaining that it took fourteen years never helped me in any way. I don't know what my soul's destiny is, and I don't know why things are the way they are. I just stayed in the game. You can keep moving forward, or not.

It should also be obvious by now that my path is about more than just physical healing. Yours may be as well. And just taking medications to get past this nuisance of an illness, caused by a random insect bite, isn't what it's about. Carolyn Myss, the best-selling author and medical intuitive, has said that when illness is part of your life path, no medical intervention can heal you until you have begun to make the changes that the illness was designed to bring about.[3]

WHY I GOT BETTER

So if I was in resistance during my whole healing path, how did I get better? The reason I was able to recover is because of the extensive amount of intense emotional healing work I did on the childhood issues that caused my illness, along with all my physical treatments. But it took fourteen years because of all the resistance.

I now realize that eliminating the daily resistance you create with suffering is one of the most important parts of healing yourself. I've provided simple and effective tools to do that in this book, even though I wasn't able to use them myself. So if I could heal myself through all the resistance I was creating, imagine what you can do if you eliminate the resistance.

GETTING LOST IN TECHNOLOGY

I've been through the whole medical thing. If you start listening to all the practitioners and specialists talk about spirochetes and their invincible ability to morph, genetics, specialized blood tests, new treatments, new technologies, intravenous antibiotic titrations, cutting-edge treatments in the works, trials being done at such and such university, parasites mutating into unknown forms and laying gazillions of eggs, different types of ticks and their lifecycles, and what types of antibiotics you need to take, you will not only get overwhelmed emotionally, but you will start to believe that this is all so complex that there is no possible way you could ever get over this. That's not true. You just haven't found the key yet. All problems seem impossible until you solve them, and then they are simple. The key to this illness is healing the underlying emotional issues.

The Amazing Human Body

The human body is an amazing mechanism. All that science knows about the body is barely the tip of the iceberg. I went down so many avenues of problems you can have with this illness—physically, mentally, and emotionally. Being an engineer and listening to all the scientific jargon, I was convinced many times that there was no possible way to get better. Scientific discussions make healing seem impossible. For fourteen years, I came out of every doctor's appointment overwhelmed and depressed. I hit a seemingly impenetrable brick wall many times, only to find a miracle that got me past it. I even destroyed my gut flora and did permanent damage to my immune system. The immune system is more important than all of the physical protocols put together. I still made it out. Why? Because emotional issues are the underlying cause of physical illness. Once you start healing the emotional, the physical is easier to treat. Once the body's innate healing mechanism is allowed to move forward without all the resistance, natural treatments may be all that are needed to assist the healing process. It's not about advanced technology. People just haven't looked at emotional healing enough.

Your body has an intelligence system far beyond anyone's comprehension. There are trillions of functions going on in your body without your awareness. Breathing and digestion are just two examples of large, complex systems that function without your awareness or intention. Don't get psyched out by what the practitioners say. They mean well. They're doing the best they can, but your body can do more than they know. I spent a fortune getting over this illness. You don't have to. I did my healing in massive emotional resistance. You don't have to.

MOVING TO THE EMOTIONAL REALM

People are starting to realize that the illness diagnosis can be more harmful than the illness itself. That's because its effect is emotional. Which specialist recommends you go out and do emotional healing? Few. Instead, they recommend the latest, most powerful treatment which will blast your physical issue to bits. The only problem is that if the issue is emotionally based, you can blast it until the cows come home and it won't do much. You have to resolve the underlying emotional issues.

When the realization hits you of just how much toxic emotional energy your body is holding due to all the hurt, fear, anger, shame and guilt that you've repressed throughout your lifetime, it will become obvious to you that releasing all that toxic sludge will help your physical healing in a big way. You'll wonder why you ever thought you could heal yourself just by taking medication. This is an inside job. Isn't that empowering though? Your health will be in your hands from now on.

HEALING YOURSELF

The way to heal yourself is laid out here. Take care of your immune system, and build your gut flora. Start right away breaking down your daily resistance to emotions that works against your body's ability to heal itself. And then work on some of your long-term emotional issues. The obstacles to your healing will begin to crumble. Physical healing protocols that have not worked in the past will start to become more effective.

You should also stop treating your healing path like a nuisance that you have to endure until it's over. Trying to avoid it is resistance. This path is part of your life. It was meant to be part of your life—there's learning in it that is essential. Allow it to be what it is and start living now, even in an impaired way. I'm not downplaying how unpleasant it can be . . . I've been there. But I know resistance doesn't help. I'm just trying to say that there is more to this path than meets the eye. Joseph Campbell, mythologist and author, has said that we must be willing to let go of the life we planned, in order to have the life that's waiting for us.[4]

I've made some comments about some spiritual beliefs here and there, because that is part of my personal healing journey. However, no belief systems of any type are needed to do any of the methods suggested in this book.

I wrote this book because too many people are trapped in this illness, going around in circles in the physical healing realm seeking one new treatment after another, waiting for new technology to be invented. It's time to do something different—emotional healing. If it doesn't cost a lot of money, or any, then what do you have to lose?

There is an excellent poem called "The Power To Change," by Jeff Foster.[5] Please Google it and read it. It captures the essence of change through nonresistance in a powerful way.

[24]

Concept of Divine Will

I've heard Panache Desai say that our souls have free will choice, but once we are in human form, we have only the illusion of free will. I've heard Byron Katie say that everything happens at the right moment, not sooner nor later. Eckhart Tolle says that there are no random events, and that the causes of events are virtually infinite and connected with the whole.[1] David Hawkins says that nothing is causing anything, and that evolution and creation are one and the same thing. Evolution is just the witnessing of creation, which is ongoing.[2] The concept that our paths have been decided before we come here, or that we just play roles that the Divine asks of us, can be called divine will, predetermination, or many other names, depending on exactly how you define it.

The only person I have heard talk about this concept at length is Panache Desai. He says that our souls have free will choice, but on some level our souls have already exercised that choice before coming here. So we come here to just play out our soul's choices for the purpose of learning. We think we have free will, but it is just an illusion. Our souls exist in a place beyond time and space, yet this reality that we currently live in has linear time and space. Is this just an illusory world where we come to learn?

ILLUSIONS

It's a little tricky to wrap your mind around that. I remember reading the book *Illusions*, by Richard Bach, back in 1984. In that book the "reluctant messiah" explains to Richard why this world is an illusion. He says that space-time is a fairly primitive school. He describes a human lifetime using the analogy of a movie reel. He says you can hold a reel of film in your hands and it's all complete, start to finish, in that moment. The film exists beyond the time that it records. If you know what the movie is, you know what's in the reel of film. There's going to be drama, battles, romance, disaster, winners, and losers. But if you really want to experience the story and get caught up in it, you have to put it in a projector and let it run through the lens minute by minute, because any illusion requires space and time to be experienced.[3]

So perhaps this reality we live in is like the projector. We can take our lives, which exist beyond time and space, and load them up into this illusory world where we can play out our soul's choices in linear time for the purpose of learning soul lessons, and for the pure visceral experience of it. As humans, we have no idea what this world is or what reality exists beyond it. All we know is that we're here.

Is Your Life's Course Predetermined?

If your life is already all planned out, you really can't do anything wrong. The outcome is already determined. You'll only be able to go the way you planned to begin with. Whether you succeed or fail has already been decided. So there's no need to chastise yourself if you fail. You didn't really screw up. It was all part of the plan. It was just for the experience—no need to take it all so personally and judge yourself because of it. You just needed that lesson.

Does that mean you don't have to do anything? No, you have to do the things that are part of your soul's plan. How do you figure out what they are? Follow your guidance or your heart.

Could it all be this simple? Was this all set up before we came here? Do we have no control over the outcomes of events in our lives? I don't know what enlightened people experience that causes them to believe these things, but they all tend to say the same thing. From my vantage point, I realize that I don't know the secrets of the universe, and I can't believe something just because an enlightened person says it is so. So why bring this up? When I entertain the belief that I have no control over outcomes that have already been decided, it takes a lot of the pressure off.

LIFE ISN'T GOING THE WAY YOU WANTED

Have you ever had the sinking feeling that life isn't going the way you wanted, especially when you have a long-term illness? It wasn't supposed to be this way, right? This sinking feeling occurs because you believe you have control over outcomes. So if you're not where you should be, then it's because you're doing something wrong. So not only are you feeling bad physically, feeling like your life is slipping away, but now you're beating yourself up over the fact that you haven't fixed it yet. If we are just playing out predetermined roles, then believing we control outcomes is the greatest of human follies. Everything is happening as it should, and you are where you are supposed to be.

KICKING MYSELF FOR NOTHING

In chapter 2, I described how I rolled on the ground rather than climbing over a fence one day, and that's when I was bitten by a tick. I spent years kicking myself for that choice—fourteen years of suffering because I made that one choice. My life was ruined by an insect. The whole decade of my forties gone, my marriage gone, hundreds of thousands of dollars in medical treatments gone. And during all that time I didn't know if I would ever recover. Until 2015 I did every last bit of my healing in a state of resistance. It was like I was holding my breath until that future day when I got better and could live again. But when I entertain the belief that this was all orchestrated, perhaps even prearranged, I just stop in my tracks. Maybe it wasn't a mistake. The whole storyline of the tragedy of a ruined life, caused by an insect bite because I was too lazy to walk around the fence, suddenly stops playing in my mind. I almost laugh when I think of all the self-punishment I put myself through for something which may have been prearranged solely for a lesson.

HOW DOES THIS CHANGE OUR LIVES?

So how does the belief in divine will change the way we live our lives? Actually, life is no different either way. Whether you believe we have free will choice, or everything is predetermined, you do the best you can from your point of view. In each situation, you make choices, so this concept doesn't change how you act. Then how is it helpful? Well, I know that we choose our beliefs. We choose many without even realizing that we choose them. We hold some beliefs fiercely for years until life demonstrates they are wrong. Then we adopt new ones. I'm not sure there is any real truth in beliefs, so why not choose to entertain beliefs that serve us? When I have an important choice to make, and it feels like the fate of my world is at stake and I am paralyzed with indecision for days, I like to entertain the thought that this decision has already been decided. It takes the edge off. It's another way to come to nonresistance. Have you ever made a choice to go one way, only to find it blocked, and then you have to go the other way? Later, you find out that it was incredibly fortunate that things turned out that way. So even if you try to make the wrong choice, maybe the universe sets you back on your chosen path.

Again, I don't know the ultimate truth of this, but it's in the *entertaining* of the notion of predetermination that the resistance is released.

CAUSALITY

We like to think that when one event occurs, and then another follows, that the first event caused the second. The scientific method depends on this. But perhaps this is just the way it appears on the surface, and causality actually comes from a much deeper place. Take, for example, the gamma rays which have been reaching Earth in the last few years in order to accelerate consciousness on the planet. One of the largest gamma ray bursts ever, GRB 140419A, was spotted on April 19, 2014. This gamma ray was from a star that exploded at the edge of the universe about 12.1 billion years ago—billions of years before the earth was even formed. When you realize that the light energy from that explosion has been traveling at the speed of light (186,000 miles per second) for 12.1 billion years, and it reached the earth at the exact time it was needed to raise the consciousness of the planet, then maybe the level of causality operating in the universe is just a little beyond our grasp.[4]

The order of the universe is unfathomable. Events are not random. Whatever brought you to this place was not an accident.

[25]

Forgiveness

Forgiveness is a tricky concept in regard to healing. It is often cited as an important act in the process of healing—emotions or illnesses. And it is, when you truly forgive. People use many methods to try to make forgiveness happen; however, forgiveness only occurs when something inside of you actually lets go of an issue. There is a magical moment in the process when you just let go. Something inside you has grown so tired of holding onto the resentment toward someone or some event, that it sees no benefit in continuing. When you truly let it go, you have made a leap forward in healing. However, before that magical moment occurs, you haven't done much; you are still holding onto the issue. What can you do to truly let an issue go? You can set an intention to forgive, work through methods of forgiveness, and try to convince yourself of the reasons why you *should* let go of the issue, but that magical moment happens when it happens, and not before. You can't make it happen. Before that moment, all the forgiveness work you do is just trying to get to the end point without fully processing the emotional issues internally. You are just trying to take a shortcut. What can you do instead?

You can feel your feelings about the person or event with the method in chapter 20. If you can process the energy of the emotional issues out of your body, then at some point you will internally let go of the issue, because there is nothing left inside you to hold onto any longer. Setting the intention to forgive is good, but that alone will not get the job done. The internal work of processing the emotions so that your body no longer wants to hold the grudge is the key.

[26]

Gratitude

If you want a quick and easy way to shift into nonresistance, try feeling gratitude. It will open your heart immediately. What to feel gratitude for? Make a list. Of course, your list will contain all the things in life that you like. Nothing wrong with that, but it's kind of pedestrian. If you want to recover from a serious illness like chronic Lyme, you'll need to think outside the box. Can you stretch yourself and be grateful for things you don't like as well? If the universe is on your side, then everything in your life is here for your benefit in some way—pain, suffering, illness, joy, love, peace. If something shows up to annoy you, then there is a purpose in that. Maybe it is some reflection of you that you weren't aware of, or maybe just an emotion coming up to process out of you for the purpose of healing.

GRATITUDE FOR THINGS YOU DON'T LIKE

If you are going to do some of the deep work of digging into yourself and your emotions, then try taking this one step further. Can you be grateful for things you don't like, trusting that it is all part of the plan? This is trusting that God knows better than you what you need to experience. Haven't you had painful experiences that you later found to be deeply meaningful to your life? Can you find the gratitude up front for painful experiences without waiting years for the wisdom that will later allow you to do so? Gratitude will open your heart further into nonresistance to life, and as we have discussed, nonresistance is where your healing begins. So the more things you can feel grateful for, the better. How about being grateful for everything? This isn't easy, but resistance to life won't help you . . . I know, I tried. I have found reasons to be grateful for parasites. They taught me how to have boundaries and how to heal myself. They have taught me about the need for self-love. Everything serves a purpose. This is not a random universe.

WHAT HAS ILLNESS TAUGHT YOU?

What has illness taught you? I needed emotional healing. If my physical illness hadn't dragged me kicking and screaming into it, I would have never done it. I'm not jumping for joy over all this, having blown most of my life being miserable, but it's a start. Besides, no matter what happened in my life before now, it would still be over with now. You're trying new things here because the old ways haven't brought you healing yet. So crazy as it sounds, try gratitude for the things you've learned in illness. How about gratitude for your body? Are you down on your body because of your illness? Do you think it let you down because it's not functioning correctly? If you look back over all the emotional issues of your life and how much you've been beating the crap out of your body with negative emotions and thoughts, you can begin to realize how hard your body is working to keep you in the ballgame. When I look back at how my body held it together for me for so long, and kept me within reach of a full recovery, I'm amazed. You can't believe what your body is doing for you right now. You can say thank you to your body. It likes that. Your body hears what you think and responds to it.

The more you feel gratitude, the more the universe brings you things to be grateful for.

[27]

Summary of
Spiritual Healing

- The repetitive negative thoughts and emotions that accompany long-term illness create a huge energy of resistance which impedes your body's innate healing process.

- Moving into nonresistance clears the way for the body's innate healing ability to proceed.

- Two methods of moving into nonresistance are presented in chapters 20 and 21. One deals with feelings, the other deals with thoughts.

- The method of consciously feeling your feelings can release vibrational density due to emotional issues from your body. This method can be used to simultaneously eliminate the daily resistance you create with suffering, as well as the long-term issues which caused your illness.

- The concept of divine will can help relieve the resistance caused by trying to control outcomes. If you believe your life was meant to be the way it is, you can let go of feeling responsible for your situation and its outcome, which reduces stress.

- Gratitude can instantly shift you into nonresistance.

RESOURCES

BOOKS

- *The Astonishing Power of Emotions* (The Teachings of Abraham) - Esther and Jerry Hicks
- *Discovering Your Soul Signature* - Panache Desai
- *A New Earth, Awakening to Your Life's Purpose* - Eckhart Tolle
- *Illusions* - Richard Bach

WEBSITES

- **www.panachedesai.com** (Website has recordings of many of his programs. These provide hours of teachings and wisdom.)
- **www.abraham-hicks.com** (Website of the Abraham-Hicks organization)

CONCLUSION

[28]

Conclusion

Summary of Entire Book

- The three parts of the book represent the three issues critical to the process of healing from chronic Lyme disease: 1) maintain your gut flora and immune system, 2) resolve the long-term emotional issues which caused your illness, and 3) eliminate the resistance caused by your daily suffering which is blocking your body's ability to heal.

- If you were not breastfed as an infant, suffered childhood trauma, and did long-term courses of antibiotics, you have a significantly compromised immune system and are a good candidate for chronic illness.

- If you can treat Lyme disease with medications that do not harm gut flora, then you may be able to avoid most of the significant chronic illness issues caused by the destruction of gut flora.

- Childhood trauma can cause emotional patterns and issues which lead to illness. If the emotional issues underlying a physical illness are deep enough, then physical treatments alone will not be able to heal the illness. The underlying emotional issues which caused the illness will have to be addressed before physical healing can occur.

- The daily repetitive negative thoughts and emotions you have, due to suffering with a long-term illness, create resistance to your healing. The practice of consciously feeling your feelings without judgment can break down this resistance and clears the way for your body's innate healing process to do its job.

- While it is tempting to focus on the physical healing part of this book, the biggest acceleration to your healing can be found in the latter two parts on emotional and spiritual healing.

- If you can treat Lyme disease without harming your gut flora, work on resolving your long-term emotional issues, and live in nonresistance to your emotions during your illness, your path of healing can be greatly accelerated.

- Health involves more than going to a doctor to get medications. Healing yourself is an inside job. You are responsible for your physical and emotional health.

THE FOCUS OF YOUR HEALING PATH

The largest part of this book is on physical healing, the second largest part is on emotional healing, and the shortest part is on spiritual healing. That mirrors the length of time I spent in each phase of healing on my journey—ten years in physical, three in emotional, and one in spiritual. It may even reflect your interest in this book, with your biggest interest in physical healing, less interest in emotional healing, and little in spiritual healing. But the potential effects of the different parts of this book on your healing path are actually in reverse order. The most important thing you can do for your healing path is to move into nonresistance, as discussed in spiritual healing, and then do some work on your long-term issues in emotional healing. And of course, you will continue physical healing, because once the energy of illness has moved to the physical level, it has to be addressed on that level; however, it should not be the only focus of your healing path. If you want to eliminate the underlying causes of the illness, you will need to go into the emotional realm.

CRACKING THE FOUNDATION OF ILLNESS

If you work on nonresistance to your current emotions, and do emotional healing of the long-term issues underlying your illness, you will bring a momentum to your healing path that you have not seen before, regardless of what you do with physical healing. When the foundation starts to crack, the whole illness structure will crumble. Be patient though. This still takes time. As your healing moves forward, there may be health crises along the way that seem to be setbacks, but they are just signs of your healing moving to a higher level.

FINAL THOUGHTS

All your life, you've been going to doctors when you got sick, and that usually worked. But this time was different. You've done everything and you still can't get better. I'm sure starting a new project on emotional healing wasn't what you had in mind, but it may be what is needed. I'm not showing you an easy shortcut here, just a way out.

I believe we are here to learn lessons. If you have chronic Lyme disease, then you are on a challenging learning path. If the universe is trying to help us, then there is some point to this. This illness is not just some unfortunate tragedy that happened to us because of an insect bite. This is the soul's way of urging us to learn the lessons we came here to learn. Perhaps there were more gentle signals along the way, inviting you to learn your lessons in an easier fashion, but you didn't get the hint. I didn't catch on, despite decades of depression and difficult relationships. So the last option life has to get your attention is to hit you over the head with a club—chronic illness. So now you're here. That's alright. How could we have known better? We didn't get an instruction manual with this body. It's not easy to figure this stuff out.

There is no way out of this predicament without learning the lessons that life has brought you to this place to learn, so you might as well get started. If it were possible to get out of this with just physical healing, you would have done so by now. If physical healing modalities are not working, it's time to take your healing to a new level and get involved with your emotional issues.

I went into emotional healing because I saw that my physical healing efforts were going nowhere. I could see from the beginning that emotional healing was the way forward, and it worked. However, emotional healing turned out to be something bigger than I had anticipated, and I continue on this path now that I have healed my illness. There is no end to learning and growing.

I hope you find the keys that unlock your pathway of healing. This is your unique journey. You will have to find *your* keys, on *your* path, in *your* way. It can be done.

Works Cited

CHAPTER 2

1   Carroll M. *Lab 257*. New York: Morrow; 2004.

2   Meinig G. *Root canal cover-up*. La Mesa, CA: Price-Pottenger Nutrition Foundation; 1998.

CHAPTER 4

1   Campbell-McBride N. *Gut and Psychology Syndrome*. [Cambridge, U.K.: Medinform Pub.]; 2010, p. 37.

2   Campbell-McBride N. *Gut and Psychology Syndrome*. [Cambridge, U.K.: Medinform Pub.]; 2010, p. 39.

3   Cowden W. NUTRAMEDIX Products - *Cowden Support Program* [Internet]. Nutramedix. 2015 [cited 2015 Nov 25];Available from: http://www.nutramedix.com/store/pc /viewPrd.asp?idcategory=5&idproduct=15

4   Seaver J. Lyme Disease Resource-*Killing Protocols* [Internet]. Lymediseaseresource.com. 2015 [cited 2015 Nov 25]; Available from: http://www.lymediseaseresource.com/ Killing_Protocols.html

5   Watson B, Stockton S. *Renew Your Life*. Clearwater, FL: Renew Life Press; 2002, p. 31.

6   Watson B, Stockton S. *Renew Your Life*. Clearwater, FL: Renew Life Press; 2002, p. 40.

7   Plummer, N. *Online videos*. 2014. Found at: *http://www.modernhcp.com/probiotics-learning-center/*

8   van Nood E, Vrieze A, Nieuwdorp M et al. *Duodenal Infusion of Donor Feces for Recurrent Clostridium difficile.* New England Journal of Medicine 2013;368(5):407-415.

9   Clark H. *Ascaris & Tapeworms* [Internet]. Drclark.net. 2015 [cited 2015 Nov 22]; Available from: http://www.drclark.net/the-essentials/beginners/parasites/ascaris-a-tapeworms 2

10   Mercola J. *There Is NO Safe Level of Using Mercury Dental Fillings (Amalgam)* [Internet]. Mercola.com. 2015 [cited 2015 Dec 7]; Available from: http://articles.mercola.com/sites/articles/archive/2015/05/09/mercury-dental-fillings.aspx

11   Nunnally S. *Dr. Nunnally Shares New Information on the Toxicity Levels of Modern Day Root Canals* [Internet]. YouTube. 2015 [cited 2015 Nov 23]; Available from: https://www.youtube.com/watch?v=BoWWXzJuuRY

12   Price W. *Home - Weston A Price* [Internet]. Weston A Price. 2015 [cited 2015 Nov 23]; Available from: http://www.westonaprice.org/

13   Wilson R. *Tooth-Organ Acumeridian Relationships* [Internet]. Naturalworldhealing.com. 2015 [cited 2015 Nov 24]; Available from: http://www.naturalworldhealing.com/Dentalinfo/toothorganchart.htm

14   Moritz A. *The Amazing Liver and Gallbladder Flush.* [Place of publication not identified]: Enter-Chi Wellness Press; 2005. p. 106.

15   Chang J. *SensibleHealth.Com: Nourish Your Body, Don't Medicate It* [Internet]. Sensiblehealth.com. 2015 [cited 2015 Nov 23]; Available from: http://www.sensiblehealth.com/LiverGallbladderFlush.xhtml

16   Wareham L. *Traditional Chinese Medicine Organ Times* [Internet]. Naturopathic By Nature. 2013 [cited 2015 Dec 17]; Available from: http://www.naturopathicbynature.com/traditional-chinese-medicine-organ-times/

17   Mercola J. *The Awful Truth About Eating Grains* [Internet]. Mercola.com. 2015 [cited 2015 Nov 27]; Available from: http://articles.mercola.com/sites/articles/archive/2008/01/02/truth-about-eating-grains.aspx

18   Mercola J, Pearsall K. *Sweet Deception*. Nashville, TN: Nelson Books; 2006.

19   Rossiter R, MacDonald S. *Overcoming Repetitive Motion Injuries the Rossiter Way*. Oakland, CA: New Harbinger Publications; 1999.

20   von Pohl G. *Geopathic Lines - Geopathic Stress Dowsing | Positive Energy* [Internet]. Positiveenergy.ie. 2015 [cited 2015 Nov 27]; Available from: http://www.positiveenergy.ie/research-on-geopathic-stress

CHAPTER 6

1   Miller A. *The Drama of the Gifted Child*. New York: Basic Books; 2007, p. 1.

CHAPTER 7

1   Miller A. *The Drama of the Gifted Child*. New York: Basic Books; 2007, pp. 8-9.

2   New Girl. Fox: 2012, Season 1, Episode 12.

3   Miller A. *The Body Never Lies*. New York: W.W. Norton; 2005, p. 25.

CHAPTER 8

1   Felitti, V. *The Adverse Childhood Experiences Study - "Turning Gold into Lead."* Ongoing.

2   TCM. *Causes of Illness - 7 Emotions* [Internet]. Sacredlotus.com. 2015 [cited 2015 Nov 28]; Available from: http://www.sacredlotus.com/go/foundations-chinese-medicine/get/causes-illness-7-emotions

3   Miller A. *The Drama of the Gifted Child.* New York: Basic Books; 2007.

4   Miller A. *The Body Never Lies.* New York: W.W. Norton; 2005.

5   Miller A. *The Body Never Lies.* New York: W.W. Norton; 2005, p. 31.

CHAPTER 9

1   Miller A. *The Drama of the Gifted Child.* New York: Basic Books; 2007, p. 34.

2   Miller A. *The Drama of the Gifted Child.* New York: Basic Books; 2007, p. 5.

3   Miller A. *The Drama of the Gifted Child.* New York: Basic Books; 2007, p. 106.

CHAPTER 10

1   Len H. *How Dr. Hew Len healed a ward of mentally ill criminals with Ho'oponopono* [Internet]. HubPages. 2015 [cited 2015 Nov 28];Available from: http://hubpages.com/religion-philosophy/How-Dr-Hew-Len-healed-a-ward-of-mentally-ill-criminals-with-Hooponopono

CHAPTER 11

1   Crane L. *The Release Technique* [Internet]. Virginia Beach, VA: Release Technique; 2015 [cited 2015 Nov 24]. Available from: http://www.releasetechnique.com

CHAPTER 12

1   Hay L. *Heal Your Body A-Z*. Carlsbad, CA: Hay House; 1998.

CHAPTER 13

1   Tolle E. *A New Earth*. New York: Plume; 2006, p. 149.
2   Ashmun J. *Narcissistic Personality Disorder (NPD) : Traits discussed* [Internet]. Halcyon.com. 2015 [cited 2015 Nov 28]; Available from: http://www.halcyon.com/jmashmun/npd/traits.html

CHAPTER 15

1   Miller A. *The Drama of the Gifted Child*. New York: Basic Books; 2007, p. 1.

CHAPTER 19

1   Tolle E. *A New Earth*. New York: Plume; 2006, p. 58.

CHAPTER 20

1   Desai P. Panache Desai - *Discover Your Soul Signature* - Home [Internet]. Panachedesai.com. 2015 [cited 2015 Nov 29]; Available from: https://www.panachedesai.com

2 Jala¯l al-Di¯n Ru¯mi¯, Barks C. *The essential Rumi*. San Francisco, CA: Harper; 1995, p. 142.

CHAPTER 21

1 Abraham, Hicks E, Hicks J. *The Astonishing Power of Emotions*. Carlsbad, Calif.: Hay House; 2007.

2 Abraham, Hicks E, Hicks J. *The Astonishing Power of Emotions*. Carlsbad, Calif.: Hay House; 2007, p. 200.

3 Abraham, Hicks E, Hicks J. *The Astonishing Power of Emotions*. Carlsbad, Calif.: Hay House; 2007, p. 52.

4 Abraham, Hicks E, Hicks J. *The Astonishing Power of Emotions*. Carlsbad, Calif.: Hay House; 2007, p. 54.

CHAPTER 23

1 Hay L. *Heal Your Body A-Z*. Carlsbad, CA: Hay House; 1998, p. 23.

2 Cannon J. *Soul speak*. Huntsville, AR: Ozark Mountain Publishing; 2013, p. 137.

3 Myss, Caroline M. *Why People Don't Heal And How They Can*. New York: Harmony Books, 1997. Print.

4 Campbell J, Osbon D. *A Joseph Campbell companion*. New York, NY: HarperCollins; 1991, p. 18.

5 Foster J. THE POWER TO CHANGE - Jeff Foster (www.lifewithoutacentre.com) | Facebook [Internet]. Facebook.com. 2015 [cited 2015 Nov 29]; Available from: https://www.facebook.com/LifeWithoutACentre/posts/720 281108069500

CHAPTER 24

1   Tolle E. *A New Earth*. New York: Plume; 2006, p. 197.

2   Hawkins D. *David R. Hawkins on causality* [Internet]. YouTube. 2015 [cited 2015 Dec 10];Available from: https://www.youtube.com/watch?v=x_bb8mw2AlY

3   Bach R. *Illusions*. [New York]: Delacorte Press; 1977, pp. 109-11.

4   O'Callaghan J. *Light from huge explosion 12.1 billion years ago reaches Earth* [Internet]. Mail Online. 2014 [cited 2015 Dec 2];Available from: http://www.dailymail.co.uk/sciencetech/article-2649425/Huge-12-billion-year-old-explosion-space-spotted-Earth-reveal-secrets-early-universe.html

ABOUT THE AUTHOR

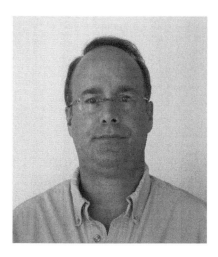

Robert Groleau has a BS in Civil Engineering and an MS in Structural Engineering, which he has used in his career as a structural engineer and consultant, specializing in bridge design, inspection, and software development.

Robert also does energy healing work in Austin, Texas—he uses a modality that clears the buildup of emotional energy, though he has studied many healing modalities. He likes to do volunteer energy healing work with veterans suffering from the chronic effects of PTSD.

Robert enjoys traveling, especially to sacred sites around the world, and many of his trips feed his interest in ancient spiritual traditions. He enjoys spending time on the lake during the hot Texan summers.

15671748R00154

Printed in Great Britain
by Amazon